T0136726

Knowledge and Representation

Knowledge
and
Representation

edited by
Albert Newen, Andreas Bartels
& Eva-Maria Jung

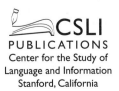

PUBLICATIONS
Center for the Study of
Language and Information
Stanford, California

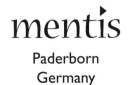

Paderborn
Germany

Library of Congress Cataloging-in-Publication Data

Knowledge and representation /
   edited by Albert Newen, Andreas Bartels & Eva-Maria Jung.

   p. cm.

Includes bibliographical references and index.

ISBN 978-1-57586-631-4 (cloth : alk. paper) –
ISBN 978-1-57586-630-7 (pbk. : alk. paper)

1. Cognition–Philosophy. 2. Philosophy and cognitive science.
3. Knowledge, Theory of. 4. Representation (Philosophy)
I. Newen, Albert. II. Bartels, Andreas, 1953- III. Jung, Eva-Maria.

BF311.K6387 2011
153–dc22

                                                                2011010799
                              CIP

Co-published with Mentis, Paderborn, Germany
ISBN 978-3-89785-749-0 (pbk. : Mentis)

∞ The acid-free paper used in this book meets the minimum requirements
of the American National Standard for Information Sciences—Permanence
of Paper for Printed Library Materials, ANSI Z39.48-1984.

CSLI was founded in 1983 by researchers from Stanford University, SRI
International, and Xerox PARC to further the research and development of
integrated theories of language, information, and computation. CSLI headquarters
and CSLI Publications are located on the campus of Stanford University.

CSLI Publications reports new developments in the study of language,
information, and computation. Please visit our web site at
http://cslipublications.stanford.edu/
for comments on this and other titles, as well as for changes
and corrections by the author and publisher.

Contents

Part II: Representation   107

Contributors

ANDREAS BARTELS
Rheinische Friedrich-Wilhelms-Universität Bonn,
Institut für Philosophie
Am Hof 1, 53113 Bonn (Germany)
✉ andreas.bartels@uni-bonn.de

WILLIAM BECHTEL
University of California, San Diego,
Department of Philosophy and Center for Chronobiology
9500 Gilman Drive, La Jolla, CA 92093-0119 (USA)
✉ bill@mechanism.ucsd.edu

ROBERT CUMMINS
University of Illinois at Urbana-Champaign,
Department of Philosophy
810 South Wright Street, Urbana, IL 61801 (USA)
✉ rcummins@illinois.edu

ANDREAS K. ENGEL
Universitätsklinikum Hamburg-Eppendorf,
Institut für Neurophysiologie und Pathophysiologie
Martinistr. 52, 20246 Hamburg (Germany)
✉ ak.engel@uke.de

EVA-MARIA JUNG
Westfälische Wilhelms-Universität Münster,
Philosophisches Seminar
Domplatz 23, 48143 Münster (Germany)
✉ eva-maria.jung@uni-muenster.de

ALBERT NEWEN
Ruhr-Universität Bochum, Institut für Philosophie
Universitätsstraße 150, 44780 Bochum (Germany)
✉ albert.newen@rub.de

GERARD O'BRIEN
University of Adelaide, School of Humanities
North Terrace, Adelaide SA 5005 (Australia)
✉ gerard.obrien@adelaide.edu.au

JONATHAN OPIE
University of Adelaide, School of Humanities
North Terrace, Adelaide SA 5005 (Australia)
✉ jonathan.opie@adelaide.edu.au

MARTIN ROTH
Drake University, Department of Philosophy and Religion
2507 University Avenue, Des Moines, IA 50316 (USA)
✉ martin.roth@drake.edu

JASON STANLEY
Rutgers University, Department of Philosophy
1 Seminary Place, New Brunswick, NJ 08901-1107 (USA)
✉ jasonintrator@gmail.com

KAI VOGELEY
Uniklinik Köln, Zentrum für Neurologie und Psychiatrie
Kerpener Str. 62, 50937 Köln (Germany)
✉ kai.vogeley@uk-koeln.de

GOTTFRIED VOSGERAU
Heinrich-Heine-Universität Düsseldorf,
Institut für Philosophie
Universitätsstr. 1, 40225 Düsseldorf (Germany)
✉ gottfried.vosgerau@uni-duesseldorf.de

GARRY YOUNG
Nottingham Trent University, School of Social Sciences
Burton Street, Nottingham, Nottinghamshire NG1 4BU (UK)
✉ garry.young@ntu.ac.uk

Preface

In this volume, we aim to present a vivid picture of main theoretical aspects of the recent debates on knowledge and representation. To this end we composed a selection of essays based on papers presented at several international workshops since 2006 on the topics "Knowing-how and Knowing-that" and "Knowledge, Representation, and Learning"; details at: http://www.wuk.uni-bonn.de/english/index_e.htm.

These workshops were part of an interdisciplinary research endeavour integrating perspectives from philosophy, psychology and neuroscience in order to reach a new understanding of knowing-how and of the natural foundations of cognitive abilities by systematically integrating recent insights in theories of representation. The organizational background of these activities have been a cooperative research project called "Knowing how and Knowing-that" and the follow-up project on "The natural foundations of cognitive and social abilities". These projects have been worked out by Andreas Bartels (Philosophy, Bonn), Albert Newen (Philosophy, Bochum), Mark May (Psychology, Hamburg), Rainer Stuhlmann-Laeisz (Philosophy, Bonn) and Kai Vogeley (Neuroscience, Köln).

We would like to thank the VolkswagenStiftung for funding these research projects and for financially supporting the workshops and the publication of this edition. We are grateful to all colleagues who accepted our invitation to contribute to this volume. Furthermore, we express our special thanks to Ramiro Glauer, Verena Gottschling, Elvira Hanisch-Kuckhoff and Ulrike Pompe who managed the practical parts of the workshop organization in a perfect way and to Jochen Faseler who did a great job in typesetting this edition.

Albert Newen, Andreas Bartels
& Eva-Maria Jung

Knowledge and Representation in the Recent Discussion: An Introduction

ANDREAS BARTELS, EVA-MARIA JUNG & ALBERT NEWEN

The volume intends to advance debates on knowledge and representation in philosophy and the cognitive sciences: the articles on knowledge focus on the understanding of knowing-how. The recent revival of the debate was mainly initiated by an article of Stanley and Williamson (2001) defending intellectualism about knowing-how, i.e., claiming that knowing-how is a species of knowing-that. The volume offers several proposals to defend and refine Ryle's classical distinction between knowing-how and knowing-that but also a clarification and defense of the Stanley and Williamson analysis.

The recent debate on representation is situated in the development of new paradigms to understand cognitive systems, i.e., extended mind, enacted mind and the dynamic systems approach. How must we change our notion of representation to account for newly discovered dimensions of cognitive systems? We reached the common ground that the classical notion of symbolic representation as developed by Fodor together with the Language of Thought hypothesis is inadequate. However, it is highly controversial whether we need only some modification of the notion of representation or its dismissal altogether. In this volume, the articles focus on new understandings of representation to account for complex human cognition as well as basic representational phenomena (like time representation in circadian clocks). But a radical counter-position denying any use of the notion of representation is also included.

The analysis of knowledge has been one of the most important projects in analytic epistemology of 20th century. Epistemologists have indefatigably tried to find an answer to the question of which conditions must be fulfilled if a subject S knows that a certain proposition p is true. Thus, the focus of the analysis is usually propositional, or factual knowledge. The so-called standard analysis defines such knowledge as "justified true belief" (JTB-analysis) and is traced back to Plato's dialogue *Theaetetus* where Socrates seeks an appropriate definition of "knowledge".

During the second half of the 20th century, however, the JTB-analysis has been attacked from different perspectives. In his seminal article *Is justified true belief knowledge?* (1963), Edmund L. Gettier has presented some putative counterexamples by which he tried to show that justified, true beliefs do not suffice for knowledge: in some cases we are inclined to ascribe the three conditions to subjects but intuitively deny that these subjects should be credited with knowledge. Being confronted with these so-called "Gettier"-cases, epistemologists have tried to modify or expand the standard analysis in order to account for the objections. A main issue had been the question of whether justification has to be understood in terms of internal reasons supporting one's true belief (Internalism), or in terms of an adequate relation to external conditions in which one's true belief is grounding (Externalism). Innumerous new definitions of knowledge have been explored after Gettier, but no one reached a broad consensus, and so we still lack a new classical analysis that could adequately replace the traditional JTB-analysis.

Moreover, the methodologies on which the JTB-analysis is grounded have also been questioned during the second half of the 20th century. For example, Edward Craig (1999) argued that the traditional analysis neglects pragmatic forces of our everyday notion of knowledge—the purposes of how we use it—and has to be replaced by what he calls a "pragmatic theory of knowledge" aiming at a "conceptual synthesis" based on the notion of reliable sources of information. By focusing on the "state of nature" Craig draws an analogy between the concept of knowledge and other concepts used in practical philosophy. Crispin Sartwell (1991, 1992), in turn, criticizes another aspect of the "JTB"-analysis: He argues that the traditional threefold analysis is inconsistent since it relies on two conditions (truth and justification) playing different roles concerning the question of epistemic goals: Whereas truth is the goal of our epistemic enterprises, justification is only a means to reach this goal or an instrument to figure out whether the goal is reached. Sartwell argues that, for this reason, a definition of knowledge that includes truth and justification as constitutive parts is illegitimate. Yet another objection against the traditional analysis is presented by Timothy Williamson (2002) who argues that knowledge is a fundamental concept that cannot be analyzed through its constitutive parts. He proposes a new knowledge-centered philosophy of mind, understanding knowledge as "the most fundamental factive mental state". In the framework of this theory, the search for an appropriate conceptual analysis of knowledge becomes superfluous. Another attack on the conceptual analysis was expressed by the so-called "Naturalized epistemology" that was firstly developed in detail by Willard Van Orman Quine (1969): Quine argues that traditional epistemology should be replaced with a naturalist project—understood as a "chapter of psychology"—focusing on the question of how our beliefs, from an empirical point of view, can be considered as reliable. Quine's arguments have been discussed controversially, leading to many other naturalized epistemologies that vary with respect to the question of the role of traditional philosophical and empirical methods for epistemological research. Yet another objection against the traditional analysis has been recently developed by so-called "experimental philosophers" (cf. Knobe and Nichols 2008): They claim that an analysis of knowledge cannot solely be developed by "armchair"-philosophy but rather has to investigate how the notion of knowledge is used in our everyday life. By focusing on investigations with philosophical laymen they aim to develop a better understanding of our folk-psychological notion of knowledge and try to show that this conflicts with the traditional analysis.

We do not have the space here to discuss all these objections the traditional analysis is confronted with in detail. Moreover, the arguments usually are connected with many other important questions of philosophy in general, for example, the question of epistemic values, or the question of the status of philosophical methodology.

This collection focuses on the notion of knowledge at the interface between traditional epistemology and the cognitive sciences. The cognitive sciences as an interdisciplinary project basically assume a broader concept of knowledge than traditional epistemology: one main assumption is that knowledge may not exclusively be acquired by human beings, but also by other cognitive systems like animals or artificial intelligent agents. Thus, if we want to develop a notion of knowledge that can also be used in cases of animals and robots we need a broader concept that does not by definition exclude these entities as candidates of knowledge. This is a reasonable move, since we have scientific explanations of the behavior of robots in AI, of animals in cognitive ethology as well as of nonlinguistic children in developmental psychology that presuppose knowledge in the explanation of the behavior. One strategy consists in widening each aspect of the classical definition of knowledge: Having a belief can be generalized to having mental representations of states of affairs, objects, events or processes which have the direction of fit that is typical of beliefs (mind-to-world). Being justified and being true is weakened to being an *adequate* representation presupposing a standard of adequacy. Thus, one core aspect of this generalization is the idea of adequate representations which may rely on different criteria of adequacy constituting different kinds of representation. Such a generalized notion of knowledge allows us to say that someone has knowledge of an entity if she has an adequate representation of it with a mind-to-world direction of fit. One consequence of this strategy is that cognitive systems can be credited with knowledge even if they do not have the capacity of propositional representations. Moreover, there are basic forms of knowledge prior to propositional representations which are grounded in nonpropositional or nonconceptual representations.

The legitimacy of such a strategy of extending the concept of knowledge has been controversially discussed in philosophy. Ryle (1949) challenged the strong focus on exclusively propositional knowledge and claimed that knowing-how marks a form of knowledge that is not reducible to knowing-that, i.e., propositional knowledge. His approach had important impacts both on traditional philosophy and empirical science such as psychology. However, Ryle's view has come under attack since, in a seminal article, Stanley and Williamson (2001) argued that knowing-how cannot be identified with abilities. Moreover, they offered a new reductive analysis of knowing-how understanding it as the knowledge that certain ways of acting are successful ones for oneself and thus they defend intellectualism concerning knowing-how. This approach led to a new discussion in different sciences. Chapters 2–5 focus on these recent discussions.

Roth and Cummins (Chapter 2) criticize Stanley and Williamson's intellectualist approach to knowing-how. More specifically, they present an argument against the methodology that is used to support intellectualism: They claim that Stanley and Williamson's analysis relies on syntactic and semantic analyses of knowledge ascriptions, i.e., on what they call an "armchair methodology", that doesn't allow for drawing consequences with respect to the discussion of knowledge-processes in cognitive science. They call Stanley and Williamson's strategy "epistemic poaching" since the latter try to support a thesis about the structure of cognitive states with linguistic methods: they argue that the semantic analysis supports the claim that a cognitive state of knowing-how has a propositional structure that therefore can be characterized in term-like sentences in a Language of Thought (LOT). Roth and Cummins try to show that scientific evidence against LOT is overwhelming, and that linguistic analyses do not have any impact on the debate about intellectualism in cognitive science since this debate is about the question of how cognitive processes are represented. They claim that both projects—the linguistic project and the project of cognitive science—should be treated as orthogonal to each other. The authors first discuss Ryle's approach to knowing-how and knowing-that and its influences on cognitive science. They claim that with the cognitive revolution intellectualism had a revolution in cognitive science (cf. Fodor 1968). This spirit can be found in the technical term "tacit knowledge" that stands for implicitly represented propositional knowledge and that is used to describe practical capacities like binding one's shoes (Fodor 1968) or the capacity of language (Chomsky 1986). From this time on, LOT became commonplace in cognitive science. Since the mid 1980s, however, the argumentative force of LOT has been doubted. Thus, many authors suggested that the exclusive propositional area is too narrow in order to capture our cognitive phenomena. Some authors argue that cognition and representation have to be understood in new terms, for example by using the notion of neural networks. Roth and Cummins then try to explain what the debates in cognitive science have to do with the discussion about knowing-how and knowing-that. According to the authors, in the context of cognitive science, intellectualism is compatible with identifying knowing-how with certain abilities, capacities, and skills. The real controversy is over the explanation of these skills, i.e., whether they are best explained on the basis of representations with propositional content or by other representations that lack such a content. Roth and Cummins present some arguments for the claim that Stanley and Williamson's analysis is irrelevant for the discussion in cognitive science. They support connectionist approaches to cognitive processes because these approaches, according to them, give us an understanding of why knowing and doing are so closely related.

In his reply to Roth and Cummins, Stanley (Chapter 3) begins with a note about terminology: Ryle introduced his terminology a long time before the debate about LOT in cognitive science got started. Thus, he does not see any reason why the word "intellectualism" should be reserved for the discussion in cognitive science. Stanley also claims that the debate about knowing-how and knowing-that is orthogonal to the question of intellectualism in cognitive science. Stanley claims that Roth and Cummins do not attack the theory Stanley and Williamson defend in general but rather focus on one part of their paper, namely, on the linguistic analysis. He claims that Stanley and Williamson do not take the linguistic analysis too much as an argument for the reduction of knowing-how to knowing-that, but rather as a positive hint. According to Stanley, legitimate objections to the account concern the question of whether there exist Gettier-cases for knowing-how, or the question of whether the linguistic analysis can be spelled out in different languages. Stanley denies that the take-home message of the new intellectualist approach is to say that LOT is plausible. Rather, they do not mention LOT at all and take their view to be entirely neutral to the question of how propositional knowledge is represented in the brain. Roth and Cummins seem to be caught in the grip of the claim that propositional attitudes can only be realized through sentence-like representations. Stanley concludes with a statement of how Stanley and Williamson's approach is of interest for cognitive science. Although they want to be neutral about the realization basis of knowing-how their view has consequences for ascriptions of knowing-how: since they take knowing-how to be essentially propositional, it is either the case that robots, animals and non-linguistic children do not possess knowing-how or that they possess propositional representations underlying their knowing-how. Here the debate on semantics seems to be connected with the cognitive debate: if it can be shown that some nonlinguistic children possess knowing-how but no concepts, and *a fortiori* no propositions, the intellectualist view is in trouble.

Garry Young (Chapter 4) presents an argument against intellectualism from a psychological point of view. He aims at demonstrating empirical evidence for the existence of a species of knowing-how that resists the intellectualist reduction. This is done via a discussion of visual agnosia. To offer additional support for the claim that knowing-how is clearly distinguishable from knowing-that he discusses the phenomenon of optical ataxia. The latter should demonstrate that exactly that part of knowing-how that remains available in cases of visual agnosia (despite a loss of relevant knowing-that) gets lost in cases of optical ataxia (despite an availability of relevant knowing-that). Before discussing visual agnosia and optical ataxia in detail, he describes Ryle's approach to knowing-how and focuses on recent objections to it developed by Snowdon. Snowdon argues for a distinction between knowing-how and the possession of some ability by discussing cases in which the ability in question is lost but intuitively the knowing-how is still present, e.g., a person who knows how to address the queen correctly but is not able to do it since being hindered by a nervous speech impediment caused by the queen's presence. *Contra* Snowdon, Young tries to present a clear case in which knowing-how and the possession of the ability merge. As a minimal condition for any knowing-how, he stresses that the candidate of a performance must rely on an intention to exclude nonintentional behavior (condition CIA). He then discusses two conditions of knowing-how to G (where G denotes an intentional action) in relation to performances: either that the actor can articulate why a performance p constitutes G or that the actor is able to experience performance p as appropriate to G. The central case of visual agnosia is introduced to illustrate that it is a case involving an intention leading systematically to successful actions but nevertheless the patient suffering from visual agnosia is not able to articulate or experience performance p as constituting G. The patient knows how to put a letter into a box only in the sense of having an ability. It seems clear that the subject should be credited with knowing-how. The complementary case of optical ataxia demonstrates a case in which the patient clearly knows that performance p would lead to G but is unable to realize a controlled performance of kind p. He is lacking the ability and thereby intuitively lacks at least one kind of knowing-how.

Jung and Newen, in Chapter 5, consider two different kinds of intellectualism: one as a semantic analysis, the other one as a cognitive or representational analysis of the mind. They claim that both kinds of intellectualism have to be attacked from different sides. Moreover, they argue that Ryle's account was misleading since he mixed these two kinds of projects. The authors deny both kinds of intellectualism: the first one by claiming that it neglects the pragmatic forces of our language use, and the second one by showing that it cannot bridge the so-called "Knowledge-Action-Gap". Furthermore, the authors sketch a new framework by abstracting from Gilbert Ryle's distinction: They argue for a distinction of two kinds of knowledge (theoretical and practical knowledge) and three so-called "knowledge"-formats that characterize ways in which information constituting knowledge can be represented. The authors try to show that these new framework allows for a better understanding of knowing-how as a common topic for philosophy and cognitive science. The argument involves the introduction of three different kinds of representation, i.e., sensorimotor representations, propositional representations and image-like representations. These distinctions mesh nicely with Young's discussion, since they allow to account for the pathological cases.

The discussion of knowing-how in this volume leads to the following observation: either we try to account for knowing-how completely in terms of propositional representations (the semantic approach) or we have to develop the distinction of Ryle into a three-fold differentiation of underlying representations (the cognitive approach). There are two different strategies to deal with the phenomenon of knowing-how. While the semantic approach intends to be neutral about questions of realization the cognitive approach is immediately leading to the search for the underlying representations.

In Part II of this edition the focus of the debate is the search for an adequate understanding of representation. As we mentioned already, there is a natural connection between the two topics: the cognitive understanding of knowing-how aims at an understanding of the underlying representations in the light of a systematic concept of representation. While the contributions of Part I of this volume tackle the question whether there exists—as Ryle has once suggested—irreducible forms of *knowing-how*, Part II accounts for a rich tradition of cognitive investigations of the mechanisms grounding elementary forms of human and non-human cognitive capacities. Some of the most impressing of those mechanisms discussed here are: regulatory systems in animals enabling them to coordinate their activities with the time of the day, human visual perception, and the neural activities underlying the social understanding of other persons' gaze. The philosophical question that is discussed in Chapters 6–10 is whether the variety of empirical accounts existing for these cognitive phenomena can be bundled by some conceptual framework, the framework of *representation*. If these phenomena turned out to be grounded in non-linguistic—or, more general, non-symbolic—representational mechanisms, a kind of unity for these phenomena would be in sight legitimating to shape the kind of *knowing-how* by means of its specific type of representational foundation. If that were true, the case for an independent status of knowing-how would be strengthened—even if the relevant forms of knowing-how could be conceptually reconstructed in form of knowing-that. Chapters 6–10 try to evaluate the prospects of such a representational foundation of knowing-how, where at least one of the contributions (Chapter 10) is severely skeptical about that prospect.

In the heydays of computational cognitive science, it was common ground that phenomena of knowledge in artificial and in natural systems have to be explained as the processing of symbolic representations. As O'Brien and Opie claim , "[c]omputation and representation were the twin foundation stones on which the whole business was based" (Chapter 6, 109). Since these days, the thesis that knowledge must be based on representations has lost its general acceptance. Representations in the sense of symbolic encodings are attacked for their being enclosed, rigid entities which are presumably unable to account for the dynamic nature of the cognitive activities of living beings unfolding in permanent interaction with their environment (see Chapter 10 for an articulation of this thesis). In addition to that, classical representationalism appears to be a child of the 'intellectualist tradition' according to which every piece of knowledge rests on a sort of rule following. Contrary to that tradition, embodied forms of knowledge have found growing attention and seem to be much more accessible by dynamical systems theory approaches than by old fashioned symbolic representations.

Nevertheless, the concept of representation seems to have more than one life: the contributions of Part II of the volume present renewed forms of the concept (far away from the symbolic tradition) and make efforts to demonstrate how these renewed variants can be applied in the understanding of highly embodied and interactive sorts of knowledge like human gaze evaluation or timekeeping control mechanisms in various animal species—sorts of knowledge that have clearly to be subsumed under the label of 'knowing-how'. Representation isn't dead; to the contrary, the authors argue, it is a necessary ingredient in the explanation of cognitive abilities. Whereas this is the general message of four of the contributions, their authors differ in their opinions as to exactly how an empirically fruitful concept of representation has to be defined. Thus, what we get from these contributions is a fair spectrum of recent approaches to representation as a tool for understanding knowledge— from strongly realist minded conceptions of representation (Chapters 6 and 7) to approaches that focus on the epistemic and methodological role of the concept (Chapters 8 and 9), to an anti-representational position requiring that the concept of representation has to be replaced with some empirically more fruitful concept (Chapter 10).

O'Brien and Opie, in their paper *Representation in Analog Computation* (Chapter 6), argue for a concept of representation which is exemplified by *analog* (versus digital) computation. The case study for analog computation is a system called 'Differential Analyzer' computing integrals by means of devices in which measurable physical quantities are made to obey mathematical relationships comparable with those existing in the original integration problem. For instance, the analog computation of the distance covered by an object in free fall does not proceed by a symbolic computation processing the differential equation for free fall, but by means of direct representation of the physical quantities occurring in free fall (as, for instance, velocity) in form of physical properties of the different constituents of the device (for instance, the angular velocity of a wheel), such that the mathematical relations between those quantities are preserved by the corresponding properties. In sum, the device as a whole behaves as a physical model of the physical process to be computed. Representation by means of physical modeling avoids one of the main objections against representational explanations: The objection is that semantical properties of representations are devoid of any causal relevance; what counts for explanation is physical causation, whereas semantical properties are at most epiphenomenal. But in the case of analog representation, the semantical properties (the contents) of the representational vehicles are fully determined by their physical properties. Thus, representational content, in that case, is not epiphenomenal, but *causally active*. Since the representational vehicles of analog representations bear semantical properties in form of real physical properties, the reality of these semantical properties cannot be disputed. Representational talk would then not be just a convenient idiom for describing a system from the perspective of its cognitive use. Representational properties would be causal properties, something that exists in nature independently from any epistemic interests and perspectives.

O'Brien and Opie claim that the "anti-representationalist movement marks a wrong turn in cognitive science. Without representation, cognitive science is bereft of its principal tool for explaining natural intelligence" (Chapter 6, 110). Indeed, if a certain cognitive behavior is modeled by means of analog representations, the causal properties of the representational vehicles which explain the occurrence of the cognitive behavior entail, at the same time, information about the objects that have to be intelligently treated by the behavior. Therefore, the explanation does not only tell some causal story about *how* the intelligent behavior comes about, but also provides insight about, *why* the behavior caused in this way is intelligent behavior, i.e., why it reflects relevant properties of the objects thus treated. The open question that still remains is as to what extent natural intelligence can indeed be modeled by means of analog representations.

William Bechtel, in his contribution *Representing Time of Day in Circadian Clocks* (Chapter 7), insists, like O'Brien and Opie, on the explanatory indispensability of representational explanations in cognitive science. His main argument for representation is instead that *mechanistic analyses* of cognitive functions require representational accounts. A mechanistic analysis, according to Bechtel, "identifies parts of a system and the operations they perform, and shows how they are organized so as to generate the phenomenon to be explained" (Chapter 7, 137). Thus, mechanistic analyses allow tackling the question of *why* a certain component of the system is present. In general, a certain component is part of the system because of its *contribution* to the generation of the phenomenon to be explained. Cognitive mechanisms, in particular, possess components the contribution of which consists in providing *information* about some external condition. If this occurs, the component represents that external condition. Even simple control systems like the Watt governor are apt to demonstrate this representation relation: Watt has inserted spindle arms in the system, because the rise and fall of the spindle arms in response to the speed of the flywheel and the angle between them is able to represent the speed, and thus the opening and closing of the valve dependent on the angle between the arms 'translates' the speed information into the appropriate control behavior of the system. This simple example illustrates what Bechtel thinks to be "a general point about representations: someone (a designer or evolution) has gone to the trouble of representing a state of affairs in a particular vehicle because that vehicle is suited for use by the consumer of that information" (Chapter 7, 138).

But perhaps this story only shows that "characterizing a component of a mechanism as a representation is useful for the person trying to understand the operation of the mechanism but that the mechanism itself has no actual representations" (Chapter 7, 140)? If that were true, then the importance of representational talk would reduce to that of a useful epistemic tool, comparable perhaps to the 'intentional systems' idiom used to simplify the explanation of purposeful behavior. The dynamical equations characterizing the operations of the Watt governor would be sufficient to explain its control function—just as dynamical equations would be sufficient to understand intelligent behavior of cognitive systems. This brings to the fore the question of the ontological status of representations. Are they really 'in the system' or are they just useful fictions?

Bechtel answers this challenge by voting for a realist conception of representation: To make the plant responsive to conditions internal or external to it, the controller must carry information about them. The informational (representational) content is in the system, it is not just 'read into it' by the interpreter. Otherwise, the controller could not perform its causal role, which consists in making the system responsive to internal or external conditions. It is important to note that this vote for realism about representation depends on the *causally active* role of representational *content*. Representational content is 'in the system' only insofar as the 'information carried by the controller' is determined by its physical properties which cause the opening or closing of the valve. The representational content must be directly 'embodied' in the causal properties of the system. Otherwise the representational properties would have some sort of ghostly existence beneath the physical properties of the system's components.

The direct embodiment of representational content in the causal properties of the representational system characterizes 'analog' representation as understood by O'Brien and Opie. Now, Bechtel, in his paper, does not explicitly propose the analog concept of representation, but favors a causal and consumer account of content in the sense of Dretske: A representational vehicle has content insofar as it carries information about its causes and that information is consumed by the system to perform some cognitive task. But in examples like the Watt governer the causal and consumer account of content is realized, for instance, by the fact that the relation between different values of the angle between the spindle arms mirrors the relation between different values of the speed of the flywheel—thus what we find is exactly analog representational content in the sense of O'Brien and Opie.

Therefore, it seems that the focus on the analog type of representation marks an important agreement between Bechtel and O'Brien and Opie concerning the conception of representational content. Bechtel, like O'Brien and Opie, defends the reality of representational content, and the reality of content can be defended in a reasonable way for the analog type of representation. If we now ask again, how far reaching this approach might be, that is, to what extent natural intelligence can be modeled by means of analog representations then the answer that Bechtel would give to that question is: "the locus of representations is within control systems, and hence [...] representation cannot be understood apart from an understanding of control systems" (Chapter 7, 140). It is thus no accident that the extended case study presented by Bechtel in the second part of his paper is devoted to a widespread type of biological control systems, namely "circadian clocks", regulating the activity of living systems by means of cellular representations of the time of day. Control systems are the natural place of representations in the biological world and the way they represent is analog representation.

Vogeley and Bartels, in their paper *The Explanatory Value of Representations in Cognitive Neuroscience* (Chapter 8), do not call into question Bechtel's representational analysis of control systems, but ask for a more comprehensive account of representational content that would be appropriate also for the contents of higher level cognitive activities of the brain that cannot be classified under the label of control systems— their case study is gaze detection and gaze evaluation as an example of social cognition. Social cognition is a challenge for a theory of representational content, since here neural systems process physical information (for example, about the duration and the direction of gaze) which is 'transformed' by that very process into social information. The point cannot be that the social aspects of the information are in any sense 'out there'; the stimuli do not bear literally 'social' properties, but only physical properties. Thus, social representational content cannot be understood by some causal account of representational content. Rather, the authors argue, the social character of some representational content is generated by means of functional connections leading from the physical input and particular neural activities processing that input, to specific forms of 'social' output in form of verbal evaluation behavior which is systematically connected to those particular neural activities.

Vogeley and Bartels infer from their case study that a general account of representational content must be a functional role account: the representational content of the neural vehicles engaged in processing the gaze behavior of other persons is determined by the functional role this activity plays in generating particular 'social' reactions to the gaze behavior. In the limiting case of detectors for some internal or external condition as they occur in Bechtel's 'control systems' this general functional role account reduces to a causal conception of content.

The functional role account does not in general assume that representational contents are 'in' the representational system. Thus it is not a realist position about representation. Nevertheless, the account takes representational contents to be explanatorily valuable. Their explanatory value is most salient, if explanation of complex, macro-level properties is at issue where these complex properties describe how a system is embedded in its environment ('entropy' would be an example from physics). Contents 'bundle' the underlying physical properties in special ways, so as to generate 'macro-level' explanations of, for instance, social behavior. In that sense, the function of representational content in explanation is that of a 'theoretical variable' which is indispensable for the generation of empirical hypotheses and predictions.

Most contributions of Part II of the volume develop their views on representation with an eye to extended empirical case studies. Vosgerau's paper *Varieties of Representation* (Chapter 9) is entirely devoted to a conceptual analysis of representation. Vosgerau's aim is to "formulate a revised functionalist theory that specifies necessary and sufficient conditions for being a representation" (Chapter 9, 187). The notion of function in this functionalist theory has to be understood in its very mathematical sense, that is, playing a functional role is to be understood as 'being an argument of some function' (cf. Chapter 9, 190). Representations are accordingly defined as substitutes of the argument-position of a (behavioral) function. For instance, if the behavior is the frog's snapping at a fly, the relevant behavioral function has perhaps 'fly in front of frog' as its argument, which can be substituted by the frog's percept of a fly. Thus, the frog's percept of a fly is a representation with respect to this behavioral function.

Since, according to Vosgerau, "a functionalist theory is not able to tell good representations from poor ones", an adequacy relation has to account for the success (or failure) of the representation. As the meaning of 'adequacy' depends on the type of representation at issue, these adequacy relations are various and therefore generate the variety of representations—in Peirce's terminology, for instance, indices are adequate representations of an object if they have been caused by that object, icons are adequate by virtue of some visual resemblance, and symbols simply by convention. In the second part of the paper, Vosgerau applies this conceptual scheme to classify sensational-, perceptual-, conceptual- and meta-representations.

An anti-representational stance is proposed in Engel's paper *Why Cognitive Neuroscience Should Adopt a "Pragmatic Stance"* (Chapter 10). Cognition, according to Engel, is not grounded in the capacity to generate 'world-models', but in a "pre-rational understanding of the world that is based on sensorimotor acquisition of real-life situations", and thus should be understood "as a form of practice itself" (Chapter 10, 211–212). Engel sees his own position as part of a 'pragmatic turn' for cognitive neuroscience as represented by the writings of, for instance Varela, Dreyfus, Clark, and O'Regan and Noë. In particular, the pragmatic turn in cognition, has appeared in the field of theories of visual perception in form of a replacement of representational accounts (e.g., Marr's theory of vision) by action-oriented accounts. While the earlier representational accounts have been inspired by the idea that the visual system consists of modules the workings of which at can be studied independently from each other and in isolation from the interaction of the body with its environment, the new action-oriented accounts take perception as arising from sensorimotor coupling by which the cognitive agent engages in the world. Neural patterns, according to this view, "'prescribe' possible actions, rather than 'describing' states of the outside world [...] their functional role in the guidance of action is what determines the 'meaning' of internal states" (Chapter 10, 226).

This action-oriented conception of the functional roles of internal states should be clearly distinguished from the traditional accounts of representational content (even from such notions like Clark's action-oriented representation) and better be expressed, according to Engel, by the new notion of a *directive*. For internal neural states, to bear specific directives, means to possess functional roles that are determined by "patterns of dynamic interactions extending through the entire cognitive system" (Chapter 10, 227).

It will be up to the reader to scrutinize how Engel's conception of directives relates to the different functional role accounts of representation presented in the preceding articles. One possible question that arises here is: How empirically "neutral" is the functional-role (in some of its version) or other accounts of representation? Is it possible, for instance, to integrate the empirical content of action-oriented theories of perception into the general scheme of a functional role account, or does this scheme by itself contain empirically relevant 'preconceptions' of cognitive capacities that exclude such inclusion?

In sum, Part II of the volume offers an overview of recent philosophical investigations on the prospects of representational accounts of knowing-how that may (or may not) be helpful to understand the various forms of non-linguistic knowledge appearing in artificial and natural systems, from analog computers and circadian clocks to social cognition. This impressive variety of cognitive phenomena will ever stimulate scientists and philosophers to search for some common conceptual ground that possibly would enable us to understand more profoundly how this variety has come into being—whether that common ground be constituted by the concept of 'representation' or some other general framework.

References

Anderson, J.R. 1996. *The Architecture of Cognition*. Lawrence Erlbaum Associates.

Anderson, J.R. 2005. *Cognitive Psychology and Its Implications*. Worth Publishers.

Audi, R. 2003. *Epistemology: A contemporary introduction to the theory of knowledge*. Routledge.

Bailer-Jones, D. 2003. When scientific models represent. *International Studies in the Philosophy of Science* 17:59–74.

Bartels, A. 2006. Defending the structural concept of representation. *Theoria* 21:7–19.

Bartels, A. and M. May. 2009. Functional role theories of representation and content explanation: with a case study from spatial cognition. *Cognitive Processing* 10:63–75.

Bechtel, W. 2001. Representations: From neural systems to cognitive systems. In W. Bechtel, P. Mandik, J. Mundale, and R. Stufflebeam, eds., *Philosophy and the Neurosciences. A Reader*, pages 332–348. Blackwell.

Bechtel, W. 2008. *Mental mechanisms: Philosophical perspectives on cognitive neuroscience*. Routledge.

Bechtel, W. and A. Abrahamsen. 1990. Beyond the excusively propositional era. *Synthese* 82:223–253.

Bechtel, W., P. Mandik, J. Mundale, and R.S. Stufflebeam, eds. 2001. *Philosophy and the Neurosciences. A Reader*. Blackwell.

BonJour, L. 2002. *Epistemology: Classic Problems and Contemporary Responses*. Rowman & Littlefield.

Brooks, R. 1991. Intelligence without representation. *Artificial Intelligence* 47:139–159.

Brown, D.G. 1970. Knowing how and knowing that, what. In O. Wood and G. Pitcher, eds., *Ryle*, pages 213–248. Macmillan.

Carr, D. 1979. The logic of knowing how and ability. *Mind* 88:394–409.

Chakravartty, A. 2009. Informational versus functional theories of scientific representation. *Synthese* 172:197–213.

Chappell, T. 2009. Plato on knowledge in the theaetetus. In E. Zalta, ed., *The Stanford Encyclopedia of Philosophy*. http://plato.stanford.edu/archives/fall2009/entries/plato-theaetetus/.

Chomsky, N. 1986. *Knowledge of Language: Its Nature, Origins, and Use*. Praeger.

Clapin, H., ed. 2002. *Philosophy of Mental Representation*. Clarendon Press.

Clark, A. and J. Toribo. 1994. Doing without representing? *Synthese* 101:401–431.

Clark, M. 1963. Knowledge and grounds: A comment on mr. gettier's paper. *Analysis* 24:46–48.

Craig, E. 1999. *Knowledge and its state of nature: An essay in conceptual synthesis*. Oxford University Press.

Cummins, R. 1989. *Meaning and mental representation*. MIT-Press.

Cummins, R. 1996. *Representations, Targets, and Attitudes*. MIT-Press.

Dretske, F. 1995. *Naturalizing the Mind*. MIT Press.

Dretske, F. 2000. *Perception, Knowledge, and Belief: Selected Essays*. Cambridge University Press.

Dretske, F. and S. Bernecker. 2000. *Knowledge. Readings in Contemporary Epistemology*. Oxford University Press.

Feldman, R. 2008. Naturalized epistemology. In E. Zalta, ed., *The Stanford Encyclopedia of Philosophy*. http://plato.stanford.edu/archives/fall2008/entries/epistemology-naturalized/.

Fodor, J. 1968. The appeal to tacit knowledge in psychological explanation. *Journal of Philosophy* 65:627–640.

Fodor, J. 1975. *The Language of Thought*. Harvard University Press.

Fodor, J. 1981. *Representations*. MIT Press.

French, S. 2003. A model-theoretic account of representation (or, i don't know much about art . . . but I know it involves isomorphism). *Philosophy of Science* 70:1472–83. abriged version.

Gärdenfors, P. 2000. *Conceptual Spaces*. MIT-Press.

Gettier, E.L. 1963. Is justified true belief knowledge? *Analysis* 23:121–123.

Goldman, A.I. 1967. A causal theory of knowing. *Journal of Philosophy* 64:357–372.

Goldman, A.I. 2000. Epistemic folkways and scientific epistemology. In G. Axtell, ed., *Knowledge, Belief, and Character. Readings in Virtue Epistemology*. Rowman & Littlefield.

Greco, J. 2010. *Achieving Knowledge. A Virtue-Theoretic Account of Epistemic Normativity*. Cambridge University Press.

Grush, R. 1995. *Emulation and Cognition*. Ph.D. thesis, University of California.

Grush, R. 2001. The architecture of representation. In W. Bechtel, P. Mandik, J. Mundale, and R. Stufflebeam, eds., *Philosophy and the Neurosciences. A Reader*, pages 349–368. Blackwell.

Hartland-Swann, J. 1958. *An Analysis of Knowing*. Allen & Unwin.

Hawley, K. 2003. Success and knowing-how. *American Philosophical Quarterly* 40:19–31.

Hornsby, J. 2007. Knowledge and abilities in action. In C. Kanzian and E. Runggaldier, eds., *Cultures. Conflict-Analysis-Dialogue. Proceedings of the 29th International Ludwig Wittgenstein-Symposium*, pages 165–180. Ontos.

Hughes, R.I.G. 1997. Models and representation. *Philosophy of Science* 64:325–336.

Keijzer, F.A. 2001. *Representation and Behavior*. MIT Press.

Kim, J. 1988. What is naturalized epistemology? In J. Tomberlin, ed., *Philosophical Perspectives 2: Epistemology*. Ridgeview.

Knobe, J.M. and S. Nichols, eds. 2008. *Experimental Philosophy*. Oxford University Press.

Koethe, J. 2002. Stanley and Williamson on knowing how. *Journal of Philosophy* 99:325–236.

Kornblith, H., ed. 1994. *Naturalizing Epistemology*. MIT Press.

Kornblith, H. 2005. *Knowledge and Its Place in Nature*. Oxford University Press.

Le Morvan, P. 2002. Is mere true belief knowledge? *Erkenntnis* 65:151–168.

Lehrer, K. 2000. *Theory of Knowledge*. Westview Press.

Lehrer, K. and T. Paxson. 1969. Knowledge: Undefeated justified true belief. *Journal of Philosophy* 66:225–237.

Markie, P. 2006. Knowing how is not knowing that. *Southwest Philosophical Review* 22:17–24.

Markman, A.B. and E. Dietrich. 2000. Expending the classical view of representation. *Trends in Cognitive Sciences* 4:470–475.

Mundy, B. 1986. On the general theory of meaningful representation. *Synthese* 67:391 437.

18 / ANDREAS BARTELS, EVA-MARIA JUNG & ALBERT NEWEN

Newen, A. and K. Vogeley. 2003. Self-representation: searching for a neural signature of self-consciousness. *Consciousness & Cognition* 12:529–543.

Nida-Rümelin, M. 2008. Qualia: The knowledge argument. In E. Zalta, ed., *The Stanford Encyclopedia of Philosophy*. http://plato.stanford.edu/archives/fall2008/entries/qualia-knowledge/.

Noë, A. 2005. Against intellectualism. *Analysis* 65:278–290.

Nozick, R. 1981. *Philosophical Explanations*. Cambridge: Harvard University Press.

O'Brien, G. and J. Opie. 1999a. A connectionist theory of phenomenal experience. *Behavioral and Brainc Sciences* 22:127–148.

O'Brien, G. and J. Opie. 1999b. Putting content into a vehicle theory of consciousness. *Behavioral and Brain Sciences* 22:175–196.

O'Brien, G. and J. Opie. 2002. Radical connectionism: Thinking with (not in) language. *Language and Communication* 22:313–329.

O'Brien, G. and J. Opie. 2006. How do connectionist networks compute? *Cognitive Processing* 7:30–41.

O'Brien, G. and J. Opie. 2009. The role of representation in computation. *Cognitive Processing* 10:53–62.

Pappas, G. 2008. Internalist vs. externalist conceptions of epistemic justification. In E. Zalta, ed., *The Stanford Encyclopedia of Philosophy*. http://plato.stanford.edu/archives/fall2008/entries/justep-intext/.

Pitt, D. 2008. Mental representation. In E. Zalta, ed., *The Stanford Encyclopedia of Philosophy*. http://plato.stanford.edu/archives/fall2008/entries/mental-representation/.

Plato. 1995. Theaetetos. In E. Duke, W. Hicken, W. Nicholl, D. Robinson, and J. Strachan, eds., *Platonis Opera*, vol. I. Oxford University Press.

Pritchard, D. 2006. *What is the Thing Called Knowledge?*. Routledge.

Pritchard, D. 2008. The value of knowledge. In E. Zalta, ed., *The Stanford Encyclopedia of Philosophy*. http://plato.stanford.edu/archives/fall2008/entries/knowledge-value/.

Quine, W.V.O. 1969. *Ontological Relativity and Other Essays*. Columbia University Press.

Rosefeldt, T. 2004. Is knowing-how simply a case of knowing-that? *Philosophical Investigations* 27:370–379.

Rowland, J. 1958. On knowing how and knowing that. *The Philosophical Review* 67:379 388.

Rumfitt, I. 2003. Savoir faire. *Journal of Philosophy* 100:158–166.

Ryle, G. 1945. Knowing how and knowing that. *Proceedings of the Aristotelian Society* 46:1–16.

Ryle, G. 1949. *The Concept of Mind*. Hutchinson.

Sartwell, C. 1991. Knowledge is merely true belief. *American Philosophical Quarterly* 28:157–165.

Sartwell, C. 1992. Why knowledge is merely true belief. *Journal of Philosophy* 89:167 180.

Shope, R.K. 2002. Conditions and analyses of knowing. In P. Moser, ed., *The Oxford Handbook of Epistemology*, pages 25–70. Oxford University Press.

Sosa, E. 2006. Reliabilism and intellectual virtue. In S. Bernecker, ed., *Reading Epistemology*, pages 80–89. Blackwell.

Sosa, E., J. Kim, and M. McGrath, eds. 2000. *Epistemology: An Anthology*. Wiley-Blackwell.

Stanley, J. and T. Williamson. 2001. Knowing how. *Journal of Philosophy* 98:411–444.

Steup, M. 2008. The analysis of knowledge. In E. Zalta, ed., *The Stanford Encyclopedia of Philosophy*. http://plato.stanford.edu/archives/fall2008/entries/knowledge-analysis/.

Suárez, M. 1999. Theories, models and representations. In L. Magnani, N. Nersessian, and P. Thagard, eds., *Model-Based Reasoning in Scientific Discovery*, pages 75–83. Kluwer.

Suárez, M. 2003. Scientific representation: Against similarity and isomorphism. *International Studies in the Philosophy of Science* 17:225–244.

Suárez, M. 2004. An inferential conception of scientific representation. *Philosophy of Science* 71:767–779.

Suppes, P. 1961. A comparison of the meaning and uses of models in mathematics and the empirical sciences. In H. Freudenthal, ed., *The Concept and the Role of the Model in Mathematics and Natural and Social Sciences*, pages 163–177. Reidel.

Swoyer, C. 1991. Structural representation and surrogative reasoning. *Synthese* 87:449–508.

Van Fraassen, B. 2008. *Scientific Representation: Paradoxes of Perspective*. Oxford University Press.

Watson, R.A. 1995. *Representational Ideas. From Plato to Patricia Churchland*. Kluwer.

Williamson, T. 2002. *Knowledge and Its Limits*. Oxford University Press.

Young, G. 2004. Bodily knowing. Re-thinking our understanding of procedural knowledge. *Philosophical Explorations* 7:37–54.

Zagzebski, L. 1996. *Virtues of the Mind*. Cambridge University Press.

Part I

Knowledge

2

Intellectualism as Cognitive Science

MARTIN ROTH & ROBERT CUMMINS

2.1 Introduction

A well entrenched view in epistemology, philosophy of mind, and cognitive science is that there is an important distinction between knowing *how* to do something and knowing *that* something is the case. According to this view, while knowing-that requires standing in a relation to a proposition, knowing-how does not; instead, knowing-how is a matter of possessing abilities, capacities, and skills, and thus constitutes a form of "nonpropositional" knowledge. However, the integrity of this distinction has been challenged, and some philosophers argue that *intellectualism*—the thesis that knowing how to do something is a matter of possessing propositional knowledge—is true. Pertinent to how this issue will be resolved, of course, are certain assumptions about the appropriate methodology for resolving it, and in this paper we argue that a certain method for establishing intellectualism is deeply suspicious. Furthermore, once we get clear about how intellectualism is understood as an *hypothesis in cognitive science*, it will become apparent that there are serious grounds for doubting the truth of intellectualism.

2.2 Against Poaching

Minimally, intellectualism is the thesis that, for any ψ, knowing how to ψ requires propositional knowledge of a way of ψ-ing. For example, according to intellectualism, if Mary knows how to tie shoes, then Mary stands in a knowledge-that relation to a proposition concerning a way of tying shoes. The most famous attack on intellectualism is due to

Knowledge and Representation.
Albert Newen, Andreas Bartels
& Eva-Maria Jung (eds.).
Copyright © 2011, CSLI Publications.

Gilbert Ryle (1949), who argued that intellectualism faces insuperable difficulties. Ryle's arguments are well known, and we will discuss some of them in the next section. Ryle's alternative to intellectualism is also well known: knowing-how is a matter of possessing abilities (multi-track dispositions to behave), not knowing that something is the case. For Ryle, such abilities include both "physical" abilities (e.g., knowing how to swim) and "mental" abilities (e.g., knowing how to multiply). Recently, however, there have been attempts to revive intellectualism, and in this paper we focus on an attempt due to Jason Stanley and Timothy Williamson (Stanley and Williamson 2001).

Stanley and Williamson offer both a criticism of the view that knowledge-how is an ability and a positive argument that knowledge-how is a species of knowledge-that. The criticism is quite simple: there are correct knowledge-how ascriptions to people who lack the abilities purportedly specified by the ascriptions. For instance, they offer the examples of a ski instructor who, though he himself cannot perform a complex stunt, may know how to perform such a stunt, and of a master piano player who loses both of her arms in a car accident (thereby losing the ability to play the piano) but is still correctly described as knowing how to play (cf. Stanley and Williamson 2001, 416). Since the thesis that knowing-how is an ability implies that these situations are impossible, and since it is intuitively plausible that there could be such an instructor and piano player, the thesis that knowledge-how is an ability is false.[1]

Turning to their positive argument, Stanley and Williamson's claim that knowledge-how is a species of knowledge-that relies on syntactic and semantic analyses of knowledge-how ascriptions. If we assume generally that the specification of truth conditions for knowledge-that ascriptions involve reference to propositions, we can clarify Stanley and Williamson's conclusion as follows: the correct specification of the truth conditions of knowledge-how ascriptions involves reference to a proposition. Furthermore, it is in virtue of the appeal to propositions in specifying the truth conditions of knowledge-how ascriptions that knowledge-how is a species of knowledge-that.

According to Stanley and Williamson, we should analyze sentences like

(1) Hannah knows how to ride a bicycle

---

[1] How conclusive are these examples? The thought underlying both cases is that if a person is presently unable to do ψ, then the person lacks the ability to ψ. Though this account of the connection between what a person is able to do and her abilities is questionable (Millikan 2000, Noë 2005), we will concede the examples for the purposes of this paper.

in the same way we analyze other sentences containing embedded questions, such as

(2) Hannah knows what to do in the case of an earthquake,

(3) Hannah knows whom to call for help.

After describing commonly accepted syntactic and semantic analyses for sentences involving embedded questions, they offer the following statement of the truth conditions for sentences like (1):

> (1) is true iff, for some contextually relevant way w which is a way for Hannah to ride a bicycle, Hannah knows that w is a way for her to ride a bicycle, under a practical mode of presentation. (cf. Stanley and Williamson 2001, 430)

Stanley and Williamson claim that if Hannah knows how to ride a bicycle, then Hannah stands in a knowledge-that relation to a Russellian proposition that contains a way of riding a bicycle as a constituent (Stanley and Williamson 2001, 427). Furthermore, Stanley and Williamson claim that the contextually relevant way w that is a constituent of a Russellian proposition can be picked out demonstratively. For example, the way which Hannah knows how to ride a bicycle may be introduced by a friend pointing to a man riding a bicycle and saying, "That is a way to ride a bicycle" (cf. Stanley and Williamson 2001, 428). Thus, Hannah's knowing how to ride a bike does not require that she be able to describe non-indexically a way for her to ride a bike. Because Stanley and Williamson show that it is possible to give an analysis of knowledge-how ascriptions using a standard account of knowledge-that ascriptions, they conclude that knowledge-how is a species of knowledge-that:

> We take our view of ascriptions of knowledge-how to be the default position. From a linguistic perspective, very little is special about ascriptions of knowledge-how. It is hard to motivate singling them out for special treatment from the rest of a family of related constructions. Our view of ascriptions of knowledge-how is the analysis reached on full consideration of these constructions by theorists unencumbered by relevant philosophical prejudices. (Stanley and Williamson 2001, 431)

On the face of it, these remarks are puzzling. As Alva Noë points out, Ryle's distinction is not intended as a thesis about the *sentences* used to attribute knowledge, but rather about the nature of knowledge itself (cf. Noë 2005). So why do Stanley and Williamson take themselves to have established intellectualism on the basis of linguistic considerations of knowledge-how ascriptions?

There is a tempting line of argument running from the semantic analysis of sentences involving "mental" terminology to conclusions about the structure of the mind. One starts, for example, with a truth-conditional analysis of belief sentences, and argues, let's say, that 'believes' is a three place relation between a believer, a proposition and a sentence in the language of thought (LOT) that expresses it (e.g., Fodor 1981). One then notes that some belief attributions are true. Since the truth condition for belief attributions requires a belief relation between a believer, a proposition and an expression in LOT, it seems that anything to which one can truly attribute beliefs must harbor psychological states with precisely that structure. And, on the assumption that the brain realizes psychological states, we get a conclusion about the structure of the brain *without having to do a single experiment!*

This is way too much for way too little. The lure of armchair neuroscience and psychology is surely too good to be true. It is what we call "epistemological poaching" (cf. Cummins 1991). A poacher is someone who hunts (or fishes) without a valid license. No sane epistemology of science will grant a neuroscience license, or a cognitive psychology license, on the basis of truth-conditional semantics and the truism that people have beliefs.

We think Stanley and Williamson are poaching when they apply their results to the debate over intellectualism. At face value, the take home message here seems to be that something like LOT and the classical program must be on the right track scientifically. The scientific evidence against LOT is not just outweighed, but trumped by some linguistically bolstered truth-conditional semantics. But the truth-conditional semantics of knowledge-how attributions, however convincingly bolstered by linguistic evidence, cannot possibly license conclusions about the viability of intellectualism in cognitive science, or about the shortcomings of its opponents. If the Stanley and Williamson analysis of knowledge ascriptions is correct (which we doubt), then we must concede the cognitive sciences may determine that those ascriptions are false. You cannot have it both ways: you cannot assume the truth of knowledge-how ascriptions, while analyzing their truth conditions in a way that prejudges substantive scientific issues.

As we will show in Section 2.4, the debate in cognitive science between advocates of intellectualism and their opponents is evidently an empirically grounded debate about what sort of functional analysis of the brain is required to explain cognitive, perceptual and motor capacities. More particularly, it is about the LOT hypothesis central to intellectualism. As that hypothesis is understood, by both its advocates and its critics, it is not an hypothesis that has implications for the proper truth-conditional semantic analysis of knowledge-how attributions. Nothing in the connectionist inspired treatment of know-how (e.g., Churchland 1989; Bechtel and Abrahamsen 1991; Haugeland 1998), for example, has any implications for the truth-conditional semantics of know-how attributions. Nor do semantic analyses of knowledge-how attributions have implications for the debate over LOT. These issues are, or should be, orthogonal to each other. If one is inclined to think that there *is* a genuine inference from a premise about the truth-conditional semantics of psychological attribution sentences to conclusions about the scientific viability of intellectualism, one should become skeptical of truth-conditional semantics. No program that licenses poaching can be right.

So, just what exactly *is* wrong with the simple move from the truth of some know-how attributions, plus the semantics of such attributions, to conclusions about intellectualism? Notice first that there obviously *is* something wrong with such arguments: they license poaching. To repeat, no sane epistemology can allow that the semantics of ordinary talk can substitute for serious neuroscience or psychology. We do not need a persuasive deconstruction of poaching arguments to know they are no good.

With that said, it seems to us that there are two possible lines of deconstruction available. The first and most radical is that truth-conditional semantics is just wrong as an account of meaning. While we have some sympathy with this idea, it doesn't really address the problem. Whether or not you believe that truth-conditional semantics is the right approach to meaning, it is hard to deny that statements have truth-conditions. Anywhere there is an overlap of vocabulary between ordinary talk on the one hand, and science on the other, truth-conditional semantics will provide a link between the substantive claims of the science and ordinary speech. That link—Davidson's Demon, we might call it, since he released it in *Truth and Meaning* (1967)—will force us either to constrain science to honor ordinary talk—to license poaching—or to constrain ordinary talk to honor science. The latter alternative, on reflection, seems obviously right. Truth conditional semantics tells us that meanings are truth-conditions. It does not, and should not, tell us the truth-values of contingent statements. We can grant Stanley and Williamson's analysis of know-how statements, but deny that it has any implications at all for cognitive science. The truth-values of our ordinary statements *should* be held hostage to the progress of science.

There is another possibility: truth-conditions, if they are to be meanings accessible from the armchair, must not go more than skin deep. They must be little more than metalanguage clones of the object language expressions under analysis. In the case of belief, for example, they should be indifferent to the differences between Dennett, Churchland, and Fodor about what beliefs actually are, if there are any. This would make semantics much less fun, of course, but it might make it more honest.[2] In the case of know-how, the lesson is that the kinds of arguments advanced by Stanley and Williamson should interest the cognitive scientist only if such arguments could bear on the debate between, e.g., connectionists and classicists; but they can't, so they shouldn't.

We do not propose to settle the issue of how semanticists should think of what they are doing so as not to engage in poaching. That, of course, is their problem. But it is a problem they must face. Semantics cannot license poaching.

2.3   Ryle on Intellectualism

Some people know how to ski, and some people who know how to ski occasionally display their knowledge on the slopes. How should we understand the relationship between knowing how to ski and particular instances of skiing? In chapter II of *The Concept of Mind* (1949), Gilbert Ryle characterizes and critiques an "intellectualist" answer to this question. According to intellectualism, as Ryle describes it, knowing how to ski requires propositional knowledge (knowledge-*that*) of ways to ski. When people act on the intention to ski, they first consult their knowledge-that and formulate a plan for action. The action itself is the output of this planning process. If we think of propositional knowledge of ways to ski as constituting a "mini-theory" of how to ski, then we can say that actions that manifest know-how are the causal consequences of a theory-driven planning process. As Ryle puts it, we first do a bit of theory and then do a bit of practice (see Ryle 1949, 29). Famously, Ryle thought intellectualism was deeply flawed. For example, he argues that intellectualism leads to an unacceptable regress: since theorizing *itself* is something we know how to do, explaining any particular instance of theorizing would require positing still *further* acts of theorizing, *ad infinitum* (Ryle 1949, 30). Hence, there has to be some knowing-how that cannot be explained in terms of knowing-that.

If intellectualism is a non-starter, what is the alternative? According to Ryle, knowledge-how is not to be found in causes, but in "capacities, skills, habits, liabilities, and bents" (Ryle 1949, 45). Exercises of

---

[2]A fair chunk of analytic metaphysics would pretty much evaporate, as well.

know-how are simply manifestations of capacities or abilities, where capacities and abilities are understood by Ryle to be dispositions "the exercises of which are indefinitely heterogeneous" (Ryle 1949, 44). For example, although Tom and Jerry may each succeed in producing the correct answer to a particular multiplication problem, if Tom is a skilled mathematician but Jerry is merely answering by rote, then Tom's behavior counts as an exercise of know-how, and Jerry's does not. The etiology of their respective behaviors is simply irrelevant. Knowing-how is a disposition, not a cause.

Ryle's argument for identifying know-how with abilities is based, in part, on how Ryle thinks we use the phrase 'know-how'. For example, consider what is involved in knowing how to play chess. Ryle writes:

> It should be noticed that the boy is not said to know how to play, if all that he can do is to recite the rules accurately. He must be able to make the required moves. But he is said to know how to play if, although he cannot recite the rules, he normally does make the permitted moves, avoid the forbidden moves and protest if his opponent makes forbidden moves. (Ryle 1949, 41)

However, it would be a mistake to conclude from this that Ryle identified know-how with dispositions to perform publicly observable behavior, for while Ryle was certainly skeptical of 'mechanistic' psychology, he did not deny the existence of operations that occur 'in the head'. For example, Ryle wasn't claiming that knowing how to multiply requires performing bits of publicly observable behavior, e.g., writing marks on paper with pencil. Rather, he emphasized that the difference between solving a problem 'in the head' and solving a problem with pencil and paper does not mark a theoretically interesting distinction, as far as the issue of *intellectualism* is concerned. To put the point another way, since the abilities that constitute know-how can be exercised "in the head", the intellectualist's distinction between theory and performance does not simply reduce to some sort of "private/public"-distinction. In addition, Ryle did not deny the existence of intellectual operations or their importance to know-how. For example, Ryle writes "the learning of all but the most unsophisticated tasks requires some intellectual capacity", which in turn requires understanding and "propositional competence" (Ryle 1949, 49). Ryle was not hostile to granting the existence of intellectual abilities (know-how), as long as this was not understood as requiring that the exercise of such abilities be preceded by some prior act of theorizing.

2.4 Intellectualism as Cognitive Science

For better or worse, in the mouths of philosophers and psychologists, the phrase 'know-how' was more or less used to refer to what Ryle said it did—abilities, capacities, and skills. Whether using 'know-how' in this way reflected actual linguistic practice simply became irrelevant—there were substantive questions about the nature and explanation of such capacities and skills, regardless of what we *called* them. Along with the cognitive revolution in psychology, however, came the revival of intellectualism. Recall that, for Ryle, intellectualism is the thesis that knowing how to ψ consists in propositional knowledge of ways to ψ, knowledge that is deployed in the course of generating ψ-behavior, and when Chomsky (1959) showed that Skinner's behaviorism was inadequate to explain language acquisition, intellectualism became a compelling *empirical hypothesis*—children possess innate knowledge of rules of grammar (knowledge-*that*), and this knowledge allows children to formulate, test, and confirm a *tacit theory* of English, a theory whose application (in part) explains their linguistic performance.

Since it was central to the cognitive revolution that much of human and animal behavior *is* best explained in terms of the deployment of propositional knowledge, if cognitive psychology had any chance at succeeding, Ryle needed to be wrong. An early attempt to refute Ryle can be found in Jerry Fodor's paper *The Appeal to Tacit Knowledge in Psychological Explanation* (1968). In this paper, Fodor defends intellectualism as an account of mental competences, which Fodor identified with abilities (e.g., the ability to play chess, the ability to speak Latin). To give a feel for his version of intellectualism, Fodor begins his paper by inviting the reader to take seriously the following explanation of how we tie our shoes:

> There is a little man who lives in one's head. The little man keeps a library. When one acts upon the intention to tie one's shoes, the little man fetches down a volume entitled *Tying One's Shoes*. The volume says such things as: "Take the left free end of the shoelace in the left hand. Cross the left free end of the shoelace over the right free end of the shoelace ...", etc. When the little man reads the instruction 'take the left free end of the shoelace in the left hand', he pushes a button on a control panel. The button is marked 'take the left free end of a shoelace in the left hand'. When depressed, it activates a series of wheels, cogs, levers, and hydraulic mechanisms. As a causal consequence of the functioning of these mechanisms, one's left hand comes to seize the appropriate end of the shoelace. Similarly, *mutatis mutandis*, for the rest of the instructions. The instructions end with the word 'end'. When the little man reads the word 'end', he returns

the book of instructions to his library. That is the way we tie our shoes. (Fodor 1968, 63)

According to this explanation, shoe tying behavior is mediated by internal processes that employ "propositions, maxims, or instructions" (Fodor 1968, 76) regarding shoe tying, and Fodor urges us to take seriously the hypothesis that a whole host of motor, perceptual, and cognitive abilities are best explained in this way. Moreover, Fodor argues that this hypothesis yields an intellectualist account of know-how: knowing how to do something consists in having an ability whose exercise has the right kind of *etiology*: "If an organism knows how to X, then nothing is a simulation of the behavior of the organism which fails to provide an answer to the question 'How do you X?' " (Fodor 1968, 75). In other words, the ability to ψ constitutes knowing how to ψ only if the causal processes that generate ψ-ing behavior represent a way to ψ. In the shoe tying example, the organism *knows how* to tie shoes since a representation of a way to tie shoes is part of the process that generates shoe tying behavior.

As Fodor was quick to acknowledge, the sorts of representations that are involved in his story about shoe tying are not usually, if ever, consciously available to the person tying her shoes. Rather, such knowledge is *tacit*, and 'tacit knowledge' is first and foremost "a theoretical term in psychology" (Fodor 1968, 76). Thus, if the kind of intellectualism that Fodor has in mind is vindicated, it will be vindicated by psychology, not philosophy or common sense. Furthermore, as his discussion makes clear, Fodor was not really interested in whether tacit knowledge is knowledge in the justified-true-belief sense that epistemologists have in mind—what he really cared about was the cognitive resources needed to explain the host of abilities and capacities that concern psychologists.

According to Fodor, those resources include LOT and computationalism: the scheme of mental representation consists in primitive symbols that can combine to form more complex representations, and mental processes are computational processes defined over the syntactic structure of LOT expressions. On this view concepts turn out to be symbols of LOT, symbols that can combine with other symbols to form complex representations with propositional content (thoughts). Since the content of a complex representation is determined by the content of its constituents and their manner of combination in the way familiar from Tarski, LOT has a compositional semantics.[3] Successfully explaining

---

[3]Fodor and Pylyshyn (1988) give a thorough exposition and defense of this position, which they call the "classical" account of concepts.

knowing-how in terms of knowing-that thus consists in showing how the manifestation of capacities is the result of processing expressions in LOT, expressions that have propositional contents.

The explanatory strategy that Fodor develops in *Tacit Knowledge* (and the intellectualist account of know-how that comes with it) has had a tremendous impact on theorizing about the mind; indeed, we can think of the history of what John Haugeland (cf. Haugeland 1998) calls Good Old-Fashioned Artificial Intelligence (GOFAI) as the history of defending the very intellectualism that Ryle discarded. In order for such a program to succeed, however, Ryle's argument against intellectualism needed refuting. So where did Ryle go wrong? The key is in appreciating that whatever know-how is required for theorizing can eventually be explained in terms of something that is itself not an exercise of the agent's know-how. In this way, Fodor's account is an instance of *homuncular functionalism* (Dennett 1978; Lycan 1987), which is a particular instance of functional analysis (Cummins 1975). The complex capacities of a person are analyzed into simpler capacities of sub-personal systems. The capacities of the sub-personal systems are in turn analyzed into even simpler capacities until we reach capacities that require no know-how to be exercised. Fodor (1987) describes the strategy as follows:

> According to this story, intelligent behavior typically exploits a 'cognitive architecture' constituted of hierarchies of symbol processors. At the top of such a hierarchy might be a quite complex capacity: solving a problem, making a plan, uttering a sentence. At the bottom, however, are only the sorts of unintelligent operations that Turing machines can perform: deleting symbols, storing symbols, copying symbols, and the rest. Filling in the middle levels is tantamount to reducing—analyzing—an intelligent capacity into a complex of dumb ones; hence to a kind of explanation of the former ... At the very top are states which may correspond to propositional attitudes that common sense is prepared to acknowledge ... But at the bottom and middle levels there are bound to be lots of symbol-processing operations that correspond to nothing that people—as opposed to their nervous systems—ever do. (Fodor 1987, 23f.)

Returning to the example of language, why did Chomsky hypothesize that children possess a tacit *theory* of language? As Ryle pointed out, our know-how consists in our open-ended ability to satisfy criteria (e.g., our ability to produce an indefinite number of novel yet grammatically correct sentences), and Chomsky argued that the best explanation of this ability is that we possess general knowledge of the principles of language—"laws" of language, so to speak—and we apply this general knowledge when we manifest our capacities. According to the computational account sketched above, theories are sets of sentences in LOT, sentences which encode the laws or principles of the domain being cognized, and applying a theory consists in inferring conclusions about particular cases from those sentences. "At the bottom", however, the symbol manipulating capacities of the hardware will constitute neither know-how nor know-that, since everything cognitive is ultimately analyzed into something non-cognitive.

By the mid 1980s, however, many researchers in cognitive science and artificial intelligence (as well as philosophers) grew skeptical that LOT accurately describes the structure of mental representations. The emergence of connectionism and computational neuroscience brought an alternative to LOT into play, and soon it became clear that many kinds of representations, including scale models, pictures, graphs, diagrams, maps, synaptic weight configurations and partitioned activation spaces and activation vectors could be evaluated for accuracy along many, often simultaneous and competing, dimensions, but not for truth. For example, consider Paul Churchland's characterization of the motive behind eliminative materialism:

> The real motive behind eliminative materialism is the worry that the 'propositional' kinematics and 'logical' dynamics of folk psychology constitute a radically false account of the cognitive activity of humans, and of the higher animals generally. The worry is that our folk conception of how cognitive creatures represent the world (by propositional attitudes) and perform computations over those representations (by drawing sundry forms of inference from one to another) is a thorough-going misrepresentation of what really takes place inside of us. (Churchland 1992, 40)

For Churchland, however, the abandonment of the propositional attitudes does not signal the abandonment of cognition, representation, and knowledge. Rather, representation and cognition need to be understood in new terms:

> The basic idea is that the brain represents the world by means of very high-dimensional activation vectors, that is, by a pattern of activation levels across a very large population of neurons. And the brain performs computations on those representations by effecting various complex vector-to-vector transformations from one neural population to another. (Churchland 1992, 41)

How do we tie our shoes, according to Churchland? There is a massively recurrent neural network that resides in your motor cortex. Given the appropriate inputs, the weight matrix of this network induces a trajectory of activation within the hidden activation space of the network, a trajectory that represents a sequence of motor outputs appropriate for shoe-tying. Because these are motor neurons, the trajectory distinctive of shoe-tying will result in orchestrated muscle movements that constitute the act of tying one's shoes.

Put in the context of cognitive science generally, the debate between those in the GOFAI camp and those in the connectionist camp is a debate over the best explanation of the target phenomena of psychology: capacities such as speaking a language, finding one's way home, seeing depth, tying one's shoes, etc. Both camps are committed to explaining capacities and abilities in terms of intentionally characterized internal states and processes; the real disagreement is over what the form and content of internal representations must be like in order to do their explanatory work.

So what, if anything, does this have to do with intellectualism, understood as the thesis that knowing-how can be reduced to, or is a species of, knowing-that? According to both Fodor and Churchland, the debate within cognitive science does have implications for intellectualism. As we've seen, Fodor claims that his proffered explanation for how we tie our shoes supports intellectualism, since the causal explanation of shoe-tying behavior involves representations of instructions for tying shoes, instructions that provide an answer to the question "How do you tie your shoes?" For Fodor, it is in virtue of shoe-tying behavior having this sort of etiology that it is correct to say that someone 'knows-how' to tie shoes. On this point, Churchland may have no disagreement with Fodor. For example, Churchland (1989) argues that the detailed motor representations of the limb movements involved in a golf swing, the representations that subserve the ability to play golf, constitute the golfer's know-how. Insofar as we can think of the processes that generate golf-playing behavior as answering the question "How do you play golf?" there appears to be no substantive difference between Fodor and Churchland. What, then, divides them? Clearly, the disagreement is over the structure and content of the representations that produce behavior. Fodor thinks that the relevant representations are sentences in LOT, sentences that have structured propositions as their contents. Churchland thinks that the relevant representations are partitioned activation spaces, spaces that represent in the way that maps do and that are not candidates for truth-conditional analysis. Thus, if by "intellectualism" we mean merely that the explanation of ψ-ing involves representations that provide an answer to the question "How does one ψ?", then both Fodor and Churchland are intellectualists. If by "intellectualism" we mean that the relevant representations have propositional contents, then Fodor, but not Churchland, is an intellectualist.

Why do Fodor and Churchland bother discussing know-how, and how much of the cognitive science hangs on the discussion? Perhaps—though it is not likely—Fodor and Churchland think that their favored theory about the architecture of cognition in some way supports, or finds support from, the folk understanding of know-how and the truth conditional analyses of know-how ascriptions such understanding supports. If so, then we say a pox on both their houses; just as physics need not support, or find support from, the folk understanding of motion, cognitive science need not support, or find support from, the folk understanding of know-how. If we bracket this motivation for speaking in terms of 'know-how', however, then talk of 'know-how' may be rather harmless. As far as the disputes in cognitive science are concerned, everyone pretty much understands what is being asserted when someone claims that knowing-how cannot be reduced to knowing-that: the correct explanation of certain abilities will not involve processing representations with propositional contents.

Let's take stock. Practically every party to the dispute between GO-FAI and connectionism accepts that knowing-how involves the possession of abilities. Furthermore, accepting this does not depend on accepting some controversial premises about the concept of know-how; using 'know-how' to refer to abilities of a certain sort is as much a matter of stipulation as anything else. Thus, in the context of cognitive science, *intellectualism is compatible with identifying know-how with certain abilities, capacities, and skills.* The real controversy is over the explanation of skills and capacities: are they best explained in terms of representations with propositional content, or are they best explained in terms of, e.g., partitioned activations spaces and prototype points, representations that lack propositional content? The reason connectionists are often aligned with Ryle (cf. Moffett and Bengson 2007) is that they agree that we will not account for many abilities in terms of representations with propositional content (knowledge-*that*); but in so agreeing, connectionists are not embracing Ryle's identification of know-how with *mere* abilities, for connectionism accounts for abilities in terms of something "cognitive" as much as GOFAI does. For example, consider how Bechtel and Abrahamsen (1991) contrast their position with Ryle's:

> Ryle's approach to analyzing knowing-how was behavioristic; he treated this knowledge as manifest in our actions and so not to be understood in terms of something hidden and internal . . . Knowing how to perform an action consisted in a disposition to perform that action when

appropriate circumstances arose. For cognitivists, however, merely saying that someone has a disposition to behave in a certain way does not suffice; what is sought is an explanation of the internal mechanisms involved. One possibility is that intelligent dispositions may not be explainable in cognitive terms; it may have to do simply with the physiological conditions accruing in one's body. But insofar as we speak of knowing how to do these things, and of these being things we learn how to do, it seems plausible to attempt to give a cognitive account of what such knowledge consists in, that is, an account in terms of one's mental activities. (Bechtel and Abrahamsen 1991, 152f.)

What is particularly striking about this passage is that, although Bechtel and Abrahamsen are open to the possibility that capacities and skills (know-how) may be given a noncognitive explanation, calling these capacities and skills *knowledge* suggests a cognitive one; and *this* suggests that if know-how were not explained in cognitive terms, then perhaps calling these capacities and skills 'know-how' would be inappropriate. Since this is a *very* un-Rylean thing to say, why are Bechtel and Abrahamsen aligned with Ryle? Because in the context of the dispute over intellectualism in cognitive science, Bechtel and Abrahamsen are anti-intellectualists. But their anti-intellectualism is not *anti-cognitivism*, but *anti-propositionalism*. Bechtel and Abrahamsen accept that the abilities they are calling 'know-how' have a basis in mental representations and processes; they just don't think the mental representations relevant to explaining skills and capacities will look like LOT. If by intellectualism we mean simply a rejection of behaviorism, then almost everyone in cognitive science is an intellectualist.

As we've seen, however, using 'know-how' and 'know-that' to formulate claims in cognitive science may provide an occasion to poach. As such, if there are independent reasons for thinking that the intellectualist account of know-how offered by Stanley and Williamson has nothing really to do with intellectualism in cognitive science, then it might be tempting to drop the talk of 'know-how' in cognitive science—it would simply do no theoretically important work. Of course, there are such reasons. The first concerns Fodor's use of 'knowledge'. As we pointed out above, Fodor's commitment to tacit knowledge is not a commitment to knowledge in the epistemologist's sense; what he really cared about was psychological explanation and the LOT he thought psychology needed. A second—and perhaps more important—reason for thinking that Stanley and Williamson's intellectualism is irrelevant to intellectualism in cognitive science concerns the resources required for intellectualism to provide a plausible explanation of behavior. Recall Fodor's explanation of how we tie our shoes: the little man in your head fetches a *book* about tying shoes. Why a book? Because according to intellectualism, the sentence in LOT that would express the relevant Russellian proposition (the kind of proposition that Stanley and Williamson would think sufficient for know-how) has to have the same form or structure as the proposition expressed, *and nobody—not even Fodor—thinks that tokening such a sentence in LOT would come anywhere close to being sufficient for an intellectualist explanation of shoe tying.* The problem, in short, is that the science requires that the structure of the representations (e.g., LOT sentences) mirror the structure of the explanatorily relevant content (e.g., a way to tie shoes), and Stanley and Williamson's account does not deliver this. Having a sentence in LOT that contains a demonstrative (e.g., 'this') that picks out a way to tie shoes will be of no help when it comes to actually getting shoes tied since, from the perspective of the science, explanatorily relevant content cannot outstrip computational form. This, by the way, is part of the reason why getting GOFAI to succeed has proven so *hard*.

The tactic of divorcing the kind of intellectualism that Stanley and Williamson defend from intellectualism in cognitive science has its costs, however. Much of the interest in intellectualism presumably rests on the assumption that establishing intellectualism would have profound consequences for our understanding of the cognitive architecture of humans. Thus, to the extent that one insulates intellectualism from the science, a vindication of intellectualism no longer looks interesting or significant. Without such insulation, however, the arguments that Stanley and Williamson adduce in support of intellectualism are irrelevant. This is no surprise: it is simply incredible that we could establish the truth of intellectualism, understood as an hypothesis in cognitive science, on the basis of the sorts of considerations they offer.

2.5   Conclusion

Intellectualism is (or should be) a substantive hypothesis about the nature of human cognition, and anti-intellectualists are betting that the best explanation of know-how will not involve LOT and propositions (GOFAI). Furthermore, though anti-intellectualism may turn out to be false, it will not be refuted by the kinds of considerations offered by Stanley and Williamson. Looking back at Ryle through the eyes of contemporary cognitive science, we can see that perhaps Ryle's most important contribution to the philosophy of mind was his insight that there is an intimate connection between *knowing* and *doing*, and that locating the knowing in an "inner place" while locating the doing in an "outer place" could not do justice to the intimacy of that connection.

Ryle's solution, of course, was to say that the knowing *is* the doing (or the tendency to do). But there is nothing wrong with positing inner mental processes to explain capacities and skills; as the failures of GO-FAI have shown, what may be wrong is (1) thinking that the kind of knowledge that explains our capacities and skills is propositional, and (2) thinking that understanding abilities, capacities, and skills is peripheral to understanding cognition. Understood this way, the problem with conceiving of knowing and doing in terms of "inner" and "outer" has nothing really to do with traditional Cartesian dualism *per se*, since the problem arises for any account of the mind that would distinguish having the knowledge relevant to abilities from applying that knowledge. Part of the appeal of connectionism is that it offers an account of how and why knowing and doing are so intimately connected, since the knowledge relevant to know-how is in the very connection weights that sub-serve the exercise of abilities, capacities, and skills.

References

Bechtel, W. and A. Abrahamsen. 1991. *Connectionism and the Mind*. Blackwell.

Chomsky, N. 1959. Review of Skinner's "Verbal Behavior". *Language* 35:26–58.

Churchland, P.M. 1989. Knowing qualia: A reply to Jackson. In *A Neurocomputational Perspective: The Nature of Mind and the Structure of Science*. MIT Press. Reprinted in: Churchland 1998, pages 143–158.

Churchland, P.M. 1992. Activation vectors vs. propositional attitudes: How the *brain* represents reality. *Philosophy and Phenomenological Research* 52. Reprinted in: Churchland 1998, pages 39–44.

Churchland, P.M. 1998. *On the Contrary: Critical Essays, 1987–1997*. MIT Press.

Cummins, R. 1975. Functional analysis. *Journal of Philosophy* 72:741–765.

Cummins, R. 1991. Methodological reflections on belief. In R. Bogdan, ed., *Mind and Common Sense: Philosophical Essays on Common Sense Psychology*, pages 53–70. Cambridge University Press.

Davidson, D. 1967. Truth and meaning. *Synthese* 17:304–323.

Dennett, D.C. 1978. *Brainstorms: Philosophical Essays on Mind and Psychology*. MIT PRess.

Fodor, J. 1968. The appeal to tacit knowledge in psychological explanation. *Journal of Philosophy* 65:627–640.

Fodor, J. 1981. *Representations*. MIT Press.

Fodor, J. 1987. *Psychosemantics*. MIT Press.

Fodor, J. and Z. Pylyshyn. 1988. Connectionism and cognitive architecture: a critical analysis. *Cognition* 28:3–71.

Haugeland, J. 1998. *Having Thought. Essays in the Metaphysics of Mind*. Harvard University Press.

Lycan, W. 1987. *Consciousness*. MIT Press.

Millikan, R.G. 2000. *On Clear and Confused Ideas*. Cambridge University Press.

Moffett, M. and J. Bengson. 2007. Know-how and concept possession. *Philosophical Studies* 136:31–57.

Noë, A. 2005. Against intellectualism. *Analysis* 65:278–290.

Ryle, G. 1949. *The Concept of Mind*. University of Chicago Press.

Stanley, J. and T. Williamson. 2001. Knowing how. *Journal of Philosophy* 98 (8):411–444.

3

Intellectualism and the Language of Thought: A Reply to Roth and Cummins

Jason Stanley

Let us call *intellectualism* the view that knowing how to do something is a species of knowing that something is the case. The purpose of Roth and Cummins's paper *Intellectualism as Cognitive Science* in Chapter 2 of this volume is to argue against the defense of intellectualism given in Stanley and Williamson (2001). According to Roth and Cummins, intellectualism is really an

> [...] empirically grounded debate about what sort of functional analysis of the brain is required to explain cognitive, perceptual and motor capacities. More particularly, it is about the LOT [Language of Thought] hypothesis central to intellectualism. (Chapter 2, 26)

Let us call the Language of Thought hypothesis (my definition) the view that an agent can only have a propositional attitude if they have a sentence-like representation in their mind/brain that (either is or) expresses the object of that attitude. Roth and Cummins accuse Stanley and Williamson of an activity they call "epistemological poaching"— deriving the truth of "something like LOT and the classical program" from conclusions derived some "some linguistically bolstered truth-conditional semantics"(cf. Chapter 2, 26). They also argue that recent work in cognitive science undermines intellectualism. More specifically, they take theorists such as Paul Churchland to have shown that

Knowledge and Representation.
Albert Newen, Andreas Bartels
& Eva-Maria Jung (eds.).
Copyright © 2011, CSLI Publications.

representations often take the form of "scale models, pictures, graphs, diagrams, maps", in short "spaces that represent in the way that maps do", and consequently "are not candidates for truth-conditional analysis", because (according to them) map-like representations cannot be ascribed propositional contents (cf. Chapter 2, 33–34).

I begin with a note about terminology: though Ryle himself introduced the terminology well before the Language of Thought hypothesis was mooted it is not my central concern to contest Roth and Cummins's view that the word "intellectualism" should be reserved for a debate about the Language of Thought hypothesis. Roth and Cummins are free to use terminology however they like. However, the debate about whether knowing how to do something is a species of knowing-that is a debate that is relevant across a wide variety of disciplines. I prefer to use vocabulary that does not specifically target issues in the philosophy of mind, as opposed to issues in epistemology. As will emerge below, the view that knowing how to do something is a species of knowing-that is orthogonal to the debate about the Language of Thought hypothesis. One can think that knowing-how is a species of knowing-that, consistently with accepting the view that mental representation is often map-like, rather than sentence-like. Or one can think that knowing-how is a species of knowing-that, consistently with accepting the Language of Thought hypothesis.

Before I turn to Roth and Cummins's main criticism of Stanley and Williamson's account of knowing-how, I will sketch the theory they are criticizing. According to Stanley and Williamson, x knows how to F if and only if for some way w, x knows that w is a way in which x could F. This account of what it is to know how to F reflects the intuitive synonymy between (for example) the proposition *that John knows how to swim* and the proposition *that John knows in what way he could swim*. Stanley and Williamson try to stay neutral about the nature of propositions. But if propositions are anything but Fregean propositions, the account must be supplemented with an account of the relevant modes of presentation, which Stanley and Williamson call *practical* modes of presentation. To think of (say) a way of swimming under a practical mode of presentation is to have a multi-track disposition towards that way of swimming—just like, for Gareth Evans, thinking of a place under the 'here' mode of presentation is to have a multi-track disposition towards that place. That is the account of knowing how to do something presented in Stanley and Williamson's paper.

Curiously, Roth and Cummins have nothing critical to say about Stanley and Williamson's account of knowing how to do something. Instead, they target one part of Stanley and Williamson's paper. In that section, Stanley and Williamson demonstrate that their view fits easily with the most natural compositional semantics for English ascriptions of knowing how to do something. In other words, what Stanley and Williamson show is that the most natural compositional semantics for English ascriptions of knowing how to do something is one according to which they express knowing how to do something, in their sense. And surely this *is* a point in favor of their analysis of knowing how to do something. It is odd to single out *for criticism* the fact that Stanley and Williamson's favored account of knowing how to do something can quite naturally be taken to be what is expressed by English ascriptions of knowing how to do something.

Suppose one produces an analysis of knowing how to do something. Surely, it would be a worry with such an analysis if there is no correct compositional semantics of English according to which ascriptions of knowing how to do something express that analysis. If there were no plausible compositional semantics for English ascriptions of knowing-how that assigned to them one's favored analysis, then that would show that one's analysis could not possibly be what English speakers mean when they use such ascriptions. It cannot be taken as a virtue of an analysis of knowing how to do something that it is not plausibly what is meant by speakers of English when they use sentences of the form 'x knows how to F'. Conversely, it surely is a virtue of Stanley and Williamson's analysis that it fits so smoothly with independently moti- vated views of the syntax and semantics of English—views formulated by theorists with no stake at all in debates about epistemology or the philosophy of mind. Stanley and Williamson do not so much take this part of their paper as an argument for their view of knowing how to do something, as much as fending off a very serious objection—viz. that their analysis of knowing how to do something cannot plausibly be taken to be what English speakers mean to express by ascriptions of knowing how to do something.

Stanley and Williamson also take the further step of assuming their analysis to be the default position on the nature of knowing how to do something. They do so, because they see other analyses of knowing how to do something as subject to this very serious objection. Perhaps they are wrong to think that other analyses of knowing-how are subject to this very serious objection. Perhaps there is some easy semantic analysis of English ascriptions of knowing how to do something that is consistent with a quite distinct picture of the nature of knowing how to do something. But Roth and Cummins have nothing to say on this score in defense of alternative analyses of knowing how to do something. For example, they do not sketch an alternative semantics of ascriptions of knowing how to do something that assign to them an analysis distinct from Stanley and Williamson's.

Of course, to say that Stanley and Williamson take their analysis to be the default position on the nature of knowing how to do something is not to say that they take their analysis to be correct. That is why the bulk of their paper is taken up responding to other potential objections to their analysis, some as serious as the objection that the analysis cannot be plausibly taken to be what English ascriptions of knowing how to do something express. These potential objections have nothing whatever to do with the claim that the smoothest compositional semantics assigns to English ascriptions of knowing how to do something their analysis. For example, since according to Stanley and Williamson's analysis, knowing how to do something is a species of propositional knowledge, their analysis entails that knowing how to do something is subject to Gettier cases, which may seem unintuitive. By showing that none of these objections succeed, Stanley and Williamson thereby defend their analysis. In short, the strategy of Stanley and Williamson's paper is to propose an analysis of knowing how to do something, and then spend the rest of the paper defending it against potential objections. One of these objections has to do with English ascriptions of knowing how to do something, and the rest do not.

Much of the critical literature since Stanley and Williamson's paper focuses, appropriately enough, on arguing that Stanley and Williamson have not adequately responded to some of the objections to their view. For example, Ian Rumfitt argues that Stanley and Williamson's analysis is not plausibly taken to be what is expressed by ascriptions of knowing how to do something. Rumfitt argues that French ascriptions of knowing how to do something do not plausibly express Stanley and Williamson's analysis (cf. Rumfitt 2003). Since French ascriptions of knowing how to do something translate English ascriptions of knowing how to do something, there must be something wrong with Stanley and Williamson's analysis of the syntax and semantics of English ascriptions of knowing how to do something. Poston (2009) provides a general argument to show that knowing how to do something is not subject to Gettier cases. These are all legitimate strategies for challenging the claims in Stanley and Williamson's paper (I respond to these challenges and others in Stanley forthcoming).

Roth and Cummins do not provide any challenges to Stanley and Williamson's argument that their analysis does smoothly fit with the compositional semantics of English embedded questions. Neither do they provide any objections to the analysis itself. Neither do they produce an alternative analysis of knowing how to do something, and perform the difficult task of showing that it can plausibly be taken to be what is expressed by a compositional analysis of English ascriptions of knowing how to do something, one that is superior to the hypothesis about English made by Stanley and Williamson. Rather, they seem to suggest that it is a *flaw* with an analysis of knowing how to do something if it can smoothly be taken to be what is expressed by English ascriptions of knowing how to do something. Something seems amiss with the dialectic here.

Roth and Cummins accuse Stanley and Williamson of something they call "epistemological poaching". Roth and Cummins describe Stanley and Williamson's mistake as follows:

> At face-value, the take home message [of Stanley and Williamson] seems to be that something like LOT and the classical program must be on the right track scientifically. The scientific evidence against LOT is not just outweighed, but trumped by some linguistically bolstered truth-conditional semantics. But the truth-conditional semantics of knowledge-how attributions, however convincingly bolstered by linguistic evidence, cannot possibly license conclusions about the viability of intellectualism in cognitive science, or about the shortcomings of its opponents. If the Stanley and Williamson analysis of knowledge ascriptions is correct (which we doubt), then we must concede the cognitive sciences may determine that those ascriptions are false. You cannot have it both ways: you cannot assume the truth of knowledge-how ascriptions, while analyzing their truth-conditions in a way that prejudges substantive scientific issues. (Chapter 2, 26)

There is some misunderstanding here. The take home message of Stanley and Williamson cannot possibly be that the Language of Thought is correct. Stanley and Williamson make no mention of the Language of Thought. They intend their analysis to be entirely neutral on how propositional knowledge is realized in the brain. As I will argue below, they were right to do so, because their analysis is consistent with the falsity of the Language of Thought hypothesis. Finally, Stanley and Williamson might both be right in their analysis of knowing how to do something, and in their analysis of ascriptions of knowing how to do something, without any of these ascriptions being true.

Roth and Cummins appear to be ascribing to Stanley and Williamson the view that some ascriptions of knowing how to do something are true. But Stanley and Williamson could be right about knowing how to do something, even if global skepticism were true.[1] Though Stanley

---

[1] As they write, "Truth-conditional semantics tells us that meanings are truth-conditions. It does not, and should not, tell us the truth-values of contingent statements. We can grant Stanley and Williamson's analysis of know-how statements,

and Williamson are both non-skeptical epistemologists, this is no part of their claim, or their argument for their claim, that knowing how to do something is a species of knowing-that. Furthermore, suppose no scientific sense could be made out of ordinary propositional attitudes— that is, suppose there is no scientific correlate of knowledge and states implicated in it, like belief. It could still be correct that knowing how to do something is a kind of knowing-that something is the case; it is just that there would be no instances of the relation of knowing that something is the case. Stanley and Williamson's view that knowing-how is a kind of knowing-that would have the same status as the thesis that belief is a relation to a proposition, if it turns out that eliminative materialism was true. They would be descriptions of properties that had no instances (or if one is sparse about properties—descriptions that did not pick out a property). It still does not follow that knowing how to do something would not be a kind of knowing that something is the case.

Still, one might reasonably be suspicious if Stanley and Williamson's analysis of knowing how to do something, conjoined with the truth of some ascriptions of knowing how to do something, entails the Language of Thought hypothesis. For example, if one rejected the Language of Thought hypothesis, but thought that some ascriptions of knowing-how were true, one would then be led to reject Stanley and Williamson's analysis of knowing how to do something. So does Stanley and Williamson's analysis of knowing how to do something entail that "LOT and the classical program are on the right track?"

According to Stanley and Williamson, to know how to ride a bicycle is to stand in a relation to a proposition containing a way of riding a bicycle, where that way is entertained under a practical mode of presentation. Is there anything here that requires a Language of Thought?

Suppose we adopt a functionalist conception of belief, according to which, "[t]o believe that P is to be disposed to act in ways that would tend to satisfy one's desires, whatever they are, in a world in which P (together with one's other beliefs) were true" (Stalnaker 1987, 15). If the functionalist conception of belief is correct, manifesting a belief is manifesting a dispositional state. On this conception of belief, manifesting one's propositional knowledge is a matter of manifesting a dispositional state that constitutes a true belief, a state acquired (say) via a reliable source. Many philosophers (e.g., Stalnaker 1987) explicitly take such a view of propositional attitudes to be consistent with the falsity of the

---

but deny that it has any implications at all for cognitive science. The truth-values of our ordinary statements *should* be held hostage to the progress of science." (Chapter 2, 27)

Language of Thought hypothesis. Unless one accepts something like Fodor's arguments for LOT, it is hard to see why someone could have the relevant dispositions only if they had sentence-like representations.

Nor does Stanley and Williamson's appeal to practical modes of presentation entail the existence of a language of thought. Stanley and Williamson model their view of modes of presentation on Evans's account of modes of presentations of objects. According to Evans, to think of a place under a 'here' mode of presentation is to have certain dispositions essentially involving that place. To think of a place p under the "here" mode of presentation is to be (for example) disposed to take off one's coat if it is very hot at p, or to put on one's coat if it is very cold at p. Similarly, to think of an object in physical space under the 'I' mode of presentation is to have certain dispositions towards that object. One thinks of that object under the 'I' mode of presentation only if one takes one's jacket off if that object is warm, and puts it on if that object is cold, etc. Analogously, to think of a way of doing something under a practical mode of presentation is to have a multi-track disposition towards that way of doing something.

Stanley and Williamson are not hostile to the Language of Thought. But their proposal, even conjoined with the truth of some knowing-how ascriptions, does not entail the existence of a Language of Thought. If one accepts that humans can have capacities and dispositions without LOT (as Roth and Cummins do), then humans can have beliefs and other propositional attitudes without a language of thought.

More generally, it is hard to see why Roth and Cummins, who are hostile to the Language of Thought, think that a creature can have propositional attitudes only if that creature has sentence-like representations. Regarding this assumption, they write:

> By the mid 1980s, however, many researchers in cognitive science and artificial intelligence (as well as philosophers) grew skeptical that LOT accurately describes the structure of mental representations. The emergence of connectionism and computational neuroscience brought an alternative to LOT into play, and soon it became clear that many kinds of representations, including scale models, pictures, graphs, diagrams, maps, synaptic weight configurations and partitioned activation spaces and activation vectors could be evaluated for accuracy along many, often simultaneous and competing, dimensions, but not for truth. (Chapter 2, 33)

And a few paragraphs later:

> [T]he disagreement [between Fodor and Churchland] is over the structure and content of the representations that produce behavior. Fodor things that the relevant representations are sentences in LOT, sentences

that have structured propositions as their contents. Churchland thinks that the relevant representations are partitioned activation spaces, spaces that represent in the way that maps do and that are not candidates for truth-conditional analysis. Thus, if by "intellectualism" we mean merely that the explanation of ψ-ing involves representations that provide an answer to the question "How does one ψ?", then both Fodor and Churchland are intellectualists. If by intellectualism we mean that the relevant representations have propositional contents, then Fodor, but not Churchland, is an intellectualist. (Chapter 2, 34–35)

Roth and Cummins seem to be brought to the view that creatures only can have propositional attitudes if they have sentence-like representations by the thought that other kinds of representations cannot have propositional content. That is presumably why they say that "scale models, pictures, graphs, diagrams, maps, synaptic weight configurations and partitioned activation spaces and activation vectors" cannot be evaluated "for truth".

However, why would one think that a map (say) does not represent propositions? An accurate map of the United States represents the proposition that Boston is North of New York City. A picture can represent the proposition that Barack Obama is sitting down, and so forth. One would think that hostility to the Language of Thought should best take the form of a rejection of the view that propositional attitudes require it (Stalnaker 1987, Matthews 2007).

Perhaps Roth and Cummins think that maps cannot represent propositions because they think of propositions as structured as sentences are (as they write, "Fodor thinks that the relevant representations are sentences in LOT, sentences that have structured propositions as their contents"). If so, then, like Stalnaker (1987), they should conclude that propositions are not structured at all, rather than concluding that beings with only map- or picture-like representations are incapable of possessing propositional attitudes.

According to Stanley and Williamson, knowing how to do something is a kind of knowing that something is the case. Though Stanley and Williamson choose a structured proposition framework in which to implement their analysis, this is merely for the sake of perspicuity. Their analysis of knowing how to do something is perfectly consistent with taking propositions to be sets of possible worlds, rather than entities that are structured like sentences. Even if it is the case that representing structured propositions is only possible in agents or systems that have something like a Language of Thought, and humans do not have something like a Language of Thought, Stanley and Williamson's account of knowing how to do something might still very well be true.

If Stanley and Williamson's view is neutral with respect to the existence of LOT, one might worry, as Roth and Cummins do towards the end of their paper, that this undermines the interest of the view that knowing-how is a kind of knowing-that. As they write:

> Much of the interest in intellectualism presumably rests on the assumption that establishing intellectualism would have profound consequences for our understanding of the cognitive architecture of humans. Thus, to the extent that one insulates intellectualism from the science, a vindication of intellectualism no longer looks interesting or significant. (Chapter 2, 37)

What is interesting and significant varies from person to person, and no doubt what is interesting and significant for epistemologists such as Stanley and Williamson may differ from what is interesting and significant for those interested principally in cognitive architecture. Nevertheless, it is hard to see why Stanley and Williamson's view has no interest or significance for Roth and Cummins, even given the fact that it is consistent with the falsity of LOT. If one is convinced, as Roth and Cummins seem to be, that LOT does not exist, and one is also convinced that some ascriptions of knowing how to do something are true, then one will be led to the conclusion that having propositional attitudes do not require the existence of LOT. If one is convinced that animals know how to do things, then one will be led to the conclusion that animals have propositional attitudes—even such subtle ones such as propositional knowledge. Of course, another conclusion one could draw from these consequences of Stanley and Williamson's view is that no ascriptions of knowing how to do something are true. One would think that even for those solely interested in cognitive architecture, at least some of these consequences are interesting and significant.

References

Matthews, R. 2007. *The Measure of Mind: Propositional Attitudes and their Attribution*. Oxford University Press.

Poston, T. 2009. Know how to be gettiered? *Philosophy and Phenomenological Research* 79 (3):743–747.

Rumfitt, I. 2003. Savoir faire. *The Journal of Philosophy* 100:158–166.

Stalnaker, R. 1987. *Inquiry*. MIT Press.

Stanley, J. forthcoming. Knowing (how). *Noûs* .

Stanley, J. and T. Williamson. 2001. Knowing how. *Journal of Philosophy* 98 (8):411–444.

4

Irreducible Forms of Knowledge-How in Patients with Visuomotor Pathologies: An Argument against Intellectualism

GARRY YOUNG

ABSTRACT

In recent years, there has been a resurgence of interest in the distinction introduced by Ryle between knowing-that and knowing-how. The focus of the debate has centred on the legitimacy of intellectualism—which posits that all knowing-how is just a species of knowing-that—as a challenge to the Rylean dichotomy. In this chapter, I add to that debate by presenting empirical evidence supporting a case for a species of knowledge-how that resists the intellectualist's reduction (and speculate over the existence of another form). By presenting two examples of visuomotor pathology—visual agnosia (in patient DF) and optic ataxia (in patient IG)—I argue that certain actions performed by DF are knowledge-based yet fail to satisfy the criteria for knowledge-that. In addition, the deficit in performance evident in IG is a result of a lack of the same knowledge-how constitutive of DF's performance. It is therefore my contention that there exists a form of intelligent action that is able to challenge the argument for exhaustive epistemic reduction championed by intellectualism, because it constitutes a genuine instance of knowledge-how is irreducible to knowledge-that.

Knowledge and Representation.
Albert Newen, Andreas Bartels
& Eva-Maria Jung (eds.).
Copyright © 2011, CSLI Publications.

4.1 Introduction

In his 1949 book *The Concept of Mind*, Gilbert Ryle presents us with two distinct species of knowledge: knowing *that* and knowing *how*. Since that time, philosophers have argued over the legitimacy of this distinction—whether it can be sustained or whether one type of knowledge is ultimately reducible to the other[1] (see Gellner 1951, Ammerman 1956, Hartland-Swann 1956, Scott 1971, Carr 1981, Upadhyaya 1982, Williamson 2000, Hertherington 2008 for a small selection of publications on this issue). More recently, there has been a resurgence of interest in this debate, particularly in the guise of *intellectualism*—as epitomised by Stanley and Williamson (2001) and Snowdon (2003)—which denies the independence of knowing-how from knowing-that, arguing instead that all knowledge-how is simply a species of propositional knowledge. More recently still, the legitimacy of intellectualism has itself been challenged (Sgaravatti and Zardini 2008, Toribio 2008, Adams 2009, Winch 2009, Young 2009), with opponents claiming that knowledge-how cannot be reduced to propositions constitutive of knowledge-that (a position often referred to as *anti-intellectualism*).[2]

In this chapter, I present my own defence of anti-intellectualism. This takes the form of case study evidence detailing both the retained visuomotor abilities of visual agnosia patient DF and the disrupted visuomotor abilities of optic ataxia patient IG. Using these studies, I argue that there exists a species of knowledge-how that is irreducible to knowledge-that (and speculate over the existence of another). It is my contention that patients like DF are able to engage in what Ryle referred to as 'intelligent' actions—actions that can be distinguished from a mere physical ability to *G*—precisely *because* their movements are knowledge-based; but, importantly, these movements, or rather the knowledge informing them, does not meet the necessary or sufficient criteria for propositional knowledge. Conversely, patients like IG are unable to engage in certain 'intelligent' actions, not because they lack the physical capacity to *G*, but because they lack a certain species of knowledge-how which enables the act of *G*-ing to occur intentionally.

Before introducing the evidence and argument in favour of a species of irreducible knowledge-how, it is first necessary to present—albeit briefly—the intellectualist's position against which these case study examples are to be used. Much of the recent discussion on intellectualism has been in response to Stanley and Williamson (2001) (e.g., Koethe

---

[1]For a discussion on the historical roots of this distinction, see Moran (2005).

[2]See Fantl (2008) for a more detailed discussion on variations of intellectualism and anti-intellectualism.

2002, Rumfitt 2003, Rosefeldt 2004, Wallis 2008, Williams 2008). However, the focus of this discussion will centre on the comparatively neglected work of Snowdon (2003), which remains faithful to the intellectualism expressed by Stanley and Williamson. This I will do in Section 4.2.

Having outlined intellectualism, it should then be possible to systematically dismantle its alleged all encompassing nature by (i) documenting further the case for a species of knowledge-how that does not fit the criteria for propositional knowledge and (ii) showing how lacking the knowledge of how to G is not the result of an absence of propositional knowledge or even the physical capacity to G; rather, it is the consequence of a an epistemic deficit that cannot be captured in propositional form. To support this argument, in Section 4.3 I will introduce patient DF and articulate the ways in which her retained visuomotor abilities resist the intellectualist's reduction, yet still remain a legitimate species of knowledge.

I will then discuss, in Section 4.4, the role played by affordances in both capturing DF's intention to G and eliciting a form of intelligent action which, when culminating in successful G-ing, constitutes an example of irreducible knowledge-how.

In Section 4.5, I will contrast the retained abilities of DF with the deficit in visuomotor action demonstrated by optic ataxia patient IG. This deficit, I will argue, makes conspicuous (by its absence in IG) the knowledge-how that is present in DF.

Finally, I will speculate over a possible additional form of irreducible knowledge-how that may account for certain abilities retained by IG.

4.2 Intellectualism and the Conditions for Intelligent Action

According to Sgaravatti and Zardini (2008), intellectualism posits that "knowing how to do something consists in (is a species of) knowing that something is the case" (Sgaravatti and Zardini 2008, 219). Or, to paraphrase Bengson et al.'s (2009) recent presentation of intellectualism, S knows how to G iff S possesses propositional knowledge regarding G. Paul Snowdon, a recent champion of intellectualism, defends this position by challenging what he calls the *Standard View* (cf. Snowdon 2003, 2), which comprises two separate but interrelated theses.

Thesis 1 *The Disjointness Thesis.* Knowing-how does not consist in knowing that some proposition is true or that some fact obtains; knowing-how cannot be reduced to or equated with (any form of) knowledge-that.

Thesis 2 *The Capacity Thesis.* Knowing how to *G* does in fact consist in being able to *G*, in having the capacity to *G*. Knowing-how ascriptions ascribe abilities or capacities to do the mentioned action.

In opposition to Thesis 1, Snowdon points out that, when ascribing knowledge relations, we typically employ a number of different knowledge terms. Often we will ascribe to someone knowledge of *why* something is the case, or of knowing *when* or *where* something is, or *whether* or *to whom* it belongs. Yet we do not contrast these knowledge ascriptions (these "knowings-*wh*") with propositional knowledge. The reason we do not, Snowdon tells us, is simple: because knowing *when x* will occur amounts to nothing more than knowing *that x* will occur at such and such a time. Therefore, despite constituting different knowledge relations, each knowing-*wh* is ultimately a form of knowing-that: "[T]hese other 'know...to...' ascriptions neatly fit the standard treatment of them as indirect ascriptions of knowing that" (Snowdon 2003, 7).

For Snowdon, knowing-how is no different; it too should be subject to the same standard (reductive) treatment. Knowing how Theseus escaped from the labyrinth is simply a case of knowing *that* he did such and such; it is equivalent to knowing facts pertaining to his escape (namely, that he retraced his steps by following the thread he had let unwind as he entered the cave). Even knowing *how to*, which Snowdon concedes is a more performance- and less factually-based form of knowledge ascription, fails to escape the standard treatment. By knowing how to proceed, I know *that* such and such must be done (see also Brown 1971). As such, 'knowing how to' is likewise subsumed within a reductive framework of propositions demonstrating, according to Hornsby and Stanley (2005), that Ryle's dichotomy is "clearly false" (Hornsby and Stanley 2005, 113). Snowdon therefore stands resolute in his opposition to any thesis which involves "rather uncomfortably, treating 'knowing how to' as the one exception to a uniform and highly plausible treatment of all other cases" (Snowdon 2003, 8).

Examples can always be found demonstrating the reduction of knowledge-how to knowledge-that. The issue is not whether such examples exist, but whether such reduction exhausts all examples. Yet even proponents of intellectualism seem to recognise that "[t]here are certain things which we are inclined to say the agent is able to simply do" (Hornsby and Stanley 2005, 114). Lihoreau (2008) refers to the use of knowledge-how in this sense to mean "ability entailing", compared to its use in Theseus escaping from the labyrinth which he calls "ability neutral" (Lihoreau 2008, 264). Does the acknowledgement—that there are things we are able simply to do—pave the way for an irreducible form of knowing how to? In other words, is this simple act (a) knowledge-based, and (b) irreducible to propositions? Snowdon would want us to say no, and recognise instead that such an acknowledgement is in fact compatible with his challenge to Thesis 2 of the Standard View (the *Capacity Thesis*).

Snowdon disagrees with the claim that knowing how to *G* and one's capacity to *G* are necessarily connected, such that knowing how to *G* entails being able to *G* and, conversely, being able to *G* entails knowing how to *G*. Of particular interest to this chapter is the latter condition (whether being able to *G* entails knowing how to *G*). With this in mind, consider the ability possessed by the subject in the following examples, which I am willing to concede *do* demonstrate that ability and 'knowing how to' lack necessary connection. Amongst other things, our subject can sneeze, hiccup and digest food (what Snowdon refers to as *basic actions*); but would we want to claim that he knows how to sneeze, hiccup, and digest food; or that as a consequence of his able digestion knows how to excrete waste? The difference between these examples and the type of intelligent action I am proposing here is well expressed by Noë: "Digestion is not an action that a person or animal can perform; it is a process that takes place inside a person or animal" (Noë 2005, 279). Thus, someone may have excellent digestion, but we would not want to say that they are good at digesting. Demonstrating one's ability to digest is not, therefore, something one can intend or fail to intend to do; it is not constitutive of a *skill* one can express.

The presence of (or even the possibility for) intention is an important addition to our discussion on whether an irreducible form of knowledge-how exists. Intention amounts to a critical distinction between a (knowledge-based) skill which enables me to engage in acts of *G*-ing, and the physical ability I have to *G* (something I am able to do irrespective of intent).[3] The inclusion of intention is also an important means of refining Ryle's notion of intelligent action. I agree with Snowdon when he argues that to say that *A* is more intelligent than *B*, because *A* has a capacity for learning which *B* lacks, is not to say that *A* knows how to learn and *B* does not (contrary to what Ryle seems to be saying), or is able to demonstrate this knowledge-how in a more

---

[3]By using the phrase "mere physical ability", I do not intend 'ability' to be synonymous with 'mechanistic'. I recognise that 'ability' has a normative (and therefore non-physical) component, even in the case of digestion or waste excretion. There is a standard or norm, arguably shaped by evolution (in these cases) that must be met in order for an ability to be demonstrated. For an informative discussion on the differences and similarities between capacity, ability and disposition, see Millikan (2000).

accomplished way. Both A and B may know how to learn insofar as they know *that* it involves attending classes, following instructions and doing one's homework (for example). But A's greater capacity for learning is not something he can intend, or likewise B not intend. Therefore, it is not knowledge-based.

My use of Ryle's notion of intelligent action requires that the action be intentional. Such an amendment avoids, I contend, Snowdon's objection that intelligence is a capacity orthogonal to knowledge-how. Our capacity to be intelligent may vary from individual to individual, but it is not something that is governed by intention—much like our capacity to digest. In addition, although including intention may narrow the scope of what constitutes intelligent action and therefore irreducible knowledge-how, I do not accept Snowdon's criticism that the existence of a species of irreducible knowledge-how only seems plausible because of the limited examples proffered. If only one instance of intelligent action of the kind I am proposing is available, then that is still sufficient to refute the claim for an *exhaustive* reduction of all knowledge-how to knowledge-that. With the refinement of Ryle's notion of intelligent action in mind, then, an amendment to Thesis 2 is required: one that recognises the importance of intention within the constitution of intelligent action, such that if one is able to G *intentionally* then it follows that one knows how to G. Let us consider Thesis 2 in light of this amendment:

Thesis 2* Knowing how to G does in fact consist in being able to G (where G is an *intentional* act). Knowing-how ascriptions ascribe abilities to do the mentioned (intentional) action.

Unlike the original Thesis 2, Thesis 2* requires that, where G is an intentional action, knowing how to G and one's ability to G are *necessarily* connected. Proponents of intellectualism may wish to deny that the amendment evident in Thesis 2* is sufficient to establish a necessary connection between one's ability to G and one's knowledge-how. I will return to this point in Section 4.3. However, irrespective of any reservations the defender of intellectualism may have over the legitimacy of Thesis 2*, for a given intelligent action to fully challenge intellectualism, it must also satisfy Thesis 1. In other words, the knowledge-how evidenced through one's ability to intentionally G must be irreducible to propositions. To refute intellectualism, then, it is necessary to show that an alleged intelligent action p is (i) performed as an intentional means of G-ing, (ii) that performing p is informed by knowledge of how to G, (iii) that this knowledge cannot be reduced to a species of knowledge-that. In short, it is necessary for subject S to satisfy what I am calling the Conditions for Intelligent Action (CIA):

(CIA) Subject S knows how to G if S is able to perform p rather than other than p, where p is a means of intentionally G-ing, and where the act of intentionally G-ing cannot be reduced to a form of knowledge-that.

Before going on to look at evidence demonstrating that there are situations that satisfy (CIA), for the sake of clarity, let us consider other forms of 'knowing how to G' that *can* be reduced to knowledge-that, and so fail as examples of intelligent action as I am using the term. The reduction evident in the examples below will inform discussion on patients DF and IG: for it is my intention to demonstrate how certain retained visuomotor abilities of DF fail to satisfies the conditions for reduction outlined below yet do meet the requirements for (CIA).

To begin, consider Julian—a classical guitarist. Julian knows how to play the guitar. In simple terms, he is able to say what constitutes various aspects of guitar playing and what does not. In knowing how to play a C major scale, for example, Julian is able to articulate that G should be played rather than G# (and with this rather than that finger). He knows that G in this context constitutes a note of the C major scale, whereas G# does not. Julian's knowledge-how means that he is able to articulate the particulars of a given performance—he knows that certain facts pertain to appropriate guitar playing and certain facts do not. More formally, we could say that Julian satisfies the first claim to knowledge (K.C.1) below:

(K.C.1) S knows how to G if S is able to *articulate* why it is that performance p constitutes G (and 'other than p' does not).

The conditions for knowledge-how expressed through (K.C.1) are, of course, nothing more than a reformulation of the intellectualist claim that, S knows how to G if and only if S possesses a certain sort of propositional knowledge regarding G. Subject S (Julian, in this case) is able to articulate why performance p (playing a G with his second finger, rather than a G# with his third) constitutes appropriate playing of a note of the C major scale). He knows *that* this is how it should be done.

It may be that (K.C.1) is sufficient to satisfy the epistemic reduction sought by intellectualism but it is not, I contend, necessary. To illustrate, consider Juan—a flamenco guitarist from Andalucia. Juan has no formal understanding of music, yet he knows how to play the guitar, flamenco style. His knowledge-how is based simply on his experience of what he performs "sounding like flamenco". Juan's experiential content is sufficient to guide his guitar playing and, where necessary, make adjustments within a given performance (see Gonzalez-Arnal 2006). It is likely that Juan is able to articulate the particulars of his performance to a limited degree using demonstrative pronouns—the reason why *that* note was (or should be) played is because it sounds better/nicer than *this* one, for example. This forms part of his reason-giving explanation and provides what McDowell calls "appropriate standing in the space of reasons" (McDowell 1995, 881; see also McDowell 1994) and Johnson refers to as "exercises of our rationality" (Johnson 1991, 7).

Juan knows that $p_1, p_2, \ldots, p_n$ are required because this is what he experiences. Therefore, even if his experience is not articulable in propositional terms beyond demonstrative pronouns, it still constitutes a form of knowledge-that because it can be used to guide his performance towards G; it is therefore the means by which p (and not 'other than p') is expressed as most appropriate. More formally:

(K.C.2) Subject S knows how to G if S is able to *experience* performance p as appropriate to G (and, conversely, 'other than p' as inappropriate).

To satisfy this second knowledge claim, and with it the intellectualist's epistemic reduction, the subject is not required to articulate, in propositional terms (beyond demonstrative pronouns), the particulars of doing G; rather, (K.C.2) credits the subject with knowledge of how to G in virtue of the link his experience forges with intentional action. In other words, through his experience he knows that he is G-ing appropriately—by doing *this*, *this* and *this*—which, of course, is what he intended to do.

Neither (K.C.1) nor (K.C.2) challenges intellectualism. Subject S's knowledge-how regarding guitar playing is either grounded in propositions—by knowing that G should be played instead of G# in context C—or that *this* note is better than *that* one. Of course, it could be argued that what Julian and Juan know how to do is apply the *rules* of guitar playing (see Jung and Newen 2010), either as formal rules of music (in the case of Julian), or (in the case of Juan) by knowing that this note sounds nicer than this one when performing Bulerias, for example. It is this demonstration of knowledge-how that can be reduced to knowing-that. Moreover, Julian and Juan may possess knowledge-how of this kind even if they are unable to physically play the guitar (perhaps owing to some tragic accident in which their hands were damaged). Their knowledge-how appears to be independent of any ability (*qua* skill) they may possess to play the guitar, further supporting

Snowdon's rebuttal of the *Capacity Thesis*—that knowledge-how and ability are necessarily connected (see also Steel 1974).

I accept that this is the case regarding the examples of knowledge-how thus far presented. However, it is my contention that the lack of necessary connection between *these* reducible forms of knowledge and one's ability to *G* does not inevitably lead to a claim that *all* demonstrations of ability are necessarily independent of a claim to knowledge, particularly when *G* is intentionally performed. Thus, I still maintain that there exists a form of intelligent action that cannot be reduced to knowledge-that. Moreover, I also question whether articulating demonstrative pronouns is in fact necessary to satisfy (K.C.2). To illustrate, consider the sheep dog that knows how to guide the sheep into the pen. In order to satisfy (K.C.2) might experiential content alone be sufficient to guide intentional performance, irrespective of the articulation of demonstrative pronouns? In the case of Juan, might the experience of one note sounding 'nicer' than another be enough for a claim to knowledge-how?[4]

In support of this argument, I draw on the work of Bermúdez who argues for a form of non-linguistic reasoning in animals and pre-verbal infants which, in part, involves a "sensitivity to regularities in the distal environment" (Bermúdez 2007, 334): what he calls "proto-conditional reasoning" (see also Bermúdez 2003). Thus, for Bermúdez, any creature with an innate sensitivity to these regularities likewise has an innate capacity to learn; and through learning "*knows that* if the gazelles see the lion they will run away" (Bermúdez 2007, 333, my italics). Now, the knowledge-that alluded to here, Bermúdez makes clear, is not (cannot be) propositional and, as such, is not a direct challenge to the intellectualist's reduction evident in (K.C.1) and (K.C.2). Nevertheless, there is a sense in which the animal watching the events unfold between the Gazelles and lion has knowledge—based on experience—that informs its understanding of the likely outcome; thereby enabling it to predict that if the gazelles see the lion they will run away. In a similar vein, might Juan, in the absence of an understanding of even demonstrative concepts, be likewise sensitive to regularities in his environments, to the effect that he knows that by moving his fingers in such and such

---

[4]An objection to the claim that experience is sufficient to guide knowledge-based movement might be as follows: Suppose the subject experiences the notes as 'sounding nice', and therefore as appropriate, even though others judge them to be inappropriate. Under such conditions would it not in fact be legitimate to say that the subject does not know how to play the guitar? In response, consider the man who rides a bicycle by sitting backwards on the seat and pedals backwards in order to move forwards. It might be claimed that his performance is inappropriate but would we want to say, in addition, that it is not something he knows how to do?

a way across the guitar strings he will produce an appropriate sound? In short, could he not predict that the outcome of this action will be a rhythm and melody appropriate to Bulerias? If so, then he seems to possess knowledge of how to G based on information contained within his experiential content that cannot be reduced to propositions, thereby satisfying (K.C.2) and (CIA) but not the intellectualist's reduction.

The debate over the existence of knowledge-how in non-human animals and pre-verbal infants is not a new one, of course, even if we extend it to include a concept-free flamenco guitarist named Juan. It is therefore not my intention to cover old ground here. Instead, I wish to challenge intellectualism by presenting a case for knowledge-how in a concept-wielding adult that cannot be reduced to propositions. In the next section, then, I will present evidence of an intentional action, the particulars of which are neither articulable in propositional terms (as required by (K.C.1)) nor, importantly, experienced by the subject as appropriate (K.C.2), because they are not *experienced* by the subject at all. It is my view that this intelligent action amounts to a demonstration of knowing how to G that is distinct from other reducible forms of knowledge-how. In effect, it is a form of knowledge-how that meets the requirements of (CIA) whilst failing to satisfy either (K.C.1) or (K.C.2)—thereby avoiding the ambiguity evident in (K.C.2). To consider this intelligent action further, I introduce the preserved visuomotor abilities of visual agnosia patient DF.

4.3   DF: Building the Case for Intelligent Action

As a result of carbon monoxide poisoning, DF's vision was so profoundly impaired that she can no longer consciously experience objects as objects. When looking at objects, she experiences only a mixture of their colours and textures with no recognisable form. Despite this impairment, DF has retained a number of specific visuomotor abilities which have been extensively studied.[5]

In one demonstration of her retained ability, DF was asked to match the orientation of a slot positioned in front of her (which could be manoeuvred through 360°) by mirroring it with her hand (Goodale et al. 1991). Over a series of trials, in which the orientation of the slot was changed, her estimation was no better than chance (which one might expect of someone who cannot 'see' the slot). However, when instructed to place a letter-like object through the slot, her performance showed a level of accuracy comparable to that of controls. In other words, despite not being able to indicate accurately the orientation of

---

[5]For an update on research relating to DF, see Goodale and Milner (2004).

the slot with her hand (in the mirroring task), DF was nevertheless consistently able to place the 'letter' through the slot, whatever its orientation, in a manner indistinguishable from controls. Does DF *know how* to place the letter through the slot?

In considering the answer, imagine that I am present during DF's first ever performance on the postal slot task. I might be forgiven for thinking that her success was simply a case of beginner's luck. Yet even in the case of luck, I would still have to concede that she possesses the physical ability to complete the task. She is clearly able to move in the required way, irrespective of whether the outcome was fortuitous. Perhaps her success is analogous to the novice dart player who, with his first ever dart, hits the required target—the bull's eye (see Carr 1979). The novice, like DF, has the physical ability to carry out the task; but would we want to declare that hitting the bull's eye is something the novice knows how to do (and is therefore a skill he can demonstrate) even if this was something he intended to at least try to do? After all, Grego (2009) reminds us, where success is possible, we tend to distinguish between success achieved through skill and mere luck.

Unfortunately, as things stand, the conditions outlined in (CIA) do not distinguish between a successful outcome that is the product of skilled (knowledge-based) performance and one that is the result of luck. Part of (CIA) holds that performing p (where p is a means of intentionally G-ing) is a measure of knowledge-how. Therefore, if DF or the novice dart player's intention is to try to G, and in performing p they succeed in G-ing, then would we not be forced to conclude that, in successfully performing p (and avoiding performing other than p), the subject has demonstrated a certain type of knowledge-how? Not according to Hawley (2003) (see also Sosa 2009), who maintains that success *per se* is neither necessary nor sufficient for a claim to knowledge. Success is not sufficient if one succeeds only once, as was the case with the novice dart player; but, importantly, neither is repeated success necessary: for it could be the case that I know how to G even if I do not succeed in G-ing every time. After all, not even David Beckham succeeds in 'bending it like Beckham' on each occasion.[6] For Hawley, what is necessary for knowledge-how is not exhaustive success but, rather, reliable success. With this in mind, perhaps we should amend (CIA) accordingly.

---

[6] Hutto also notes that actions which exhibit knowledge-how, in the form of a certain ability (or what I would call 'skill'), do not require this ability to be "infallible" (Hutto 2005, 390).

(**CIA***) Subject S knows how to G if S is able to perform p reliably, rather than other than p, where p is a means of intentionally G-ing, and where the act of G-ing cannot be reduced to a form of knowledge-that.

Of course, it could be argued that the vast majority of us 'succeed' at breathing, or digesting food, or excreting waste: these are things we consistently do, and their success and reliability are measured against a backdrop of normative evolutionary function. But as pointed out by Noë earlier, we would be reluctant to credit ourselves with knowledge of how to perform these tasks, for they are merely examples of processes or happenings, not intentional acts. This view is echoed by Hawley when she states: "success cannot amount to knowledge-how unless intentional action is involved" (Hawley 2003, 26). However, for Hawley, in addition to the intention, to exhibit knowledge-how the subject must 'understand' (i) that she has succeeded in doing G (in other words, she must be aware that what she has done constitutes successful G-ing), and (ii) that her performance p constituted a good way of achieving the goal of doing G (she must be aware of the connection between her chosen method and the best—or at least an appropriate—method of achieving G).[7]

The extent of the subject's 'understanding' in relation to (i) and (ii) seems compatible with (K.C.1) and (K.C.2). Both my awareness of success when performing G and my awareness of the fact that my chosen method (performance p) is appropriate to achieving G are implied within each of these respective claims to knowledge. It may be that I am able to articulate this awareness (a requirement of (K.C.1)) or, instead, that I simply experience it as such (as required by (K.C.2)); either way, it seems that the species of knowledge-how that is able to satisfy Hawley's conditions likewise satisfies in some form or other at least one of these knowledge claims.

DF's success at the postal slot task is remarkably consistent, thus supporting the claim that she demonstrates reliable success. But does DF's success satisfy each of Hawley's conditions? As DF completes her performance, she is aware of the 'letter' correctly passing through the slot—thus satisfying condition (i). However, DF and patients with related pathologies, such as those suffering from blindsight (see Weiskrantz 1986, 1997), are often amazed, initially at least, by their success. A point endorsed by Grunbaum whilst discussing the performance of a blindsight patient:

---

[7]I do not wish to make condition (ii) too demanding. The subject simply needs to be aware that the method is appropriate; this appropriateness can be based on cultural norms, or be quite idiosyncratic—appropriate (as in, it works) for me.

If she has no perceptual contact with her environment, her motor behaviour, the grand level of her intentional engagement with the world,
will appear to her as unintelligible, and its success as a matter of pure
luck. (Grunbaum 2008, 251)

The fact that blindsight patients and even those suffering from visual
agnosia believe that what they are doing is simply 'guessing' suggests
that each fails to satisfy condition (ii). As they grow accustomed to
their success, however, they are less likely to attribute it to guess work
(a point I shall return to).

So is DF aware of the connection between her chosen method and
some appropriate method of achieving G? Yes, in so far as she understands that performance p is an attempt to satisfy her intention to
obey the command "Place the letter through the slot", even if, initially
at least, she considers such an attempt pointless. In other words, she
knows, generally, what is involved in posting a letter through a slot and
what is not (I *know that* I should reach forward rather than, say, lift
my hand up in the air). DF is therefore aware that her performance is
intentional in so far as it is *intended* to comply with the researcher's
request, and she knows that reaching forward is a reasonable means of
achieving this.[8] However, in light of DF's visual agnosia, the degree to
which it can be claimed that she is aware of the more specific details[9] of
the match between her chosen method and some appropriate method
of achieving G is questionable. In fact, I would go so far as to say that,
initially, she is not, nor can she be, aware of this. However, the extent
to which she can *become* aware of her success is discussed below.

We know that DF lacks conscious awareness of the position of the
slot. In what sense, then, is she able to connect her chosen method of
execution with an appropriate method of posting the letter? Her initial
sense of pointlessness would seem to indicate that she is not *aware*
of knowing how to carry out this task *qua* knowing what specifically
to do—other than knowing how to reach forward with a letter *as if*

---

[8] Apart from DF's lack of ability to consciously experience objects (as objects),
she is, of course, in all other respects 'normal'. She is aware of her condition, and
of what the researcher is asking her to do, and of the supposed mismatch between
task and alleged knowledge-how. Her initial surprise at the request is testament to
this. Therefore, however reluctant she may be (initially, at least) to perform action
p, her initiation of the action conforms to the requirements of the command, as best
she understands it. It is this compliance that makes performance p intentional, and
distinguishes it from, say, digesting food.

[9] By "more specific details", I simply mean a conscious awareness of the slot's
orientation that she will have to mirror in order to post the letter. I certainly do not
require DF to be aware of precise angles of orientation, or trajectory, which would
be beyond most (if not all) of us to articulate.

to post it. But this is not the same thing. At most it is compatible with the general awareness she has of her performance's compliance with the researcher's command (as noted above). There is no specific information contained within the command "Place-the-letter-through-the-slot" to indicate how this is to be achieved.

Perhaps DF's intention is simply to indulge the experimenter by *reaching forward* in a half-hearted attempt to post the letter. After all, DF knows how to reach forward! This knowledge-how, I accept, can be reduced to knowledge that—she knows *that* reaching forward entails doing such and such, and knows that such action complies with at least the attempt to obey the command. But knowing facts pertaining to how to reach forward does not explain her continued success on the postal-slot task. To understand why, let us allow that her intention is to do more than simply reach forward and is, instead, a genuine attempt at posting the letter. Even if this is the case, to reiterate, in terms of what DF is aware of it is not at all clear what could be informing the specifics of her performance. What awareness does she have that her chosen method matches the best (or an appropriate) method of G-ing? She cannot consciously perceive the position of the slot, so there is every reason to suspect that she has no awareness at all of the best (or an appropriate) method to use. Therefore, simply reaching forward (which is what DF initially 'felt' she was doing) even in a genuine attempt to post the letter through the slot seems inadequate to satisfy Hawley's condition (ii).

Having said that, DF and patients with related pathologies, can grow accustomed to their success. Yet even if repeated success provides DF with an air of confidence—and with it an awareness of impending success that she lacked during her initial trials—her actual performance has not altered. If we compared her early trial performances with those of the 'more confident' DF, would we want to say that *now* she knows how to post the letter through the slot whereas before she did not? DF has become aware of the success of her chosen method, thus satisfying Hawley's condition (ii); but is this awareness constitutive of newly acquired knowledge-how? It seems intuitively the case that after reflecting back on all of DF's other trials and the consistency of her performances, instead of concluding that DF now knows how to G one must accept that she already knew this. This knowledge-how was demonstrable without the awareness required by condition (ii): an awareness that I argued earlier was compatible with either (K.C.1) or (K.C.2).

What is it, then, that is informing this intelligent action? In other words, what forms the basis for this knowledge-how, such that it is independent of and irreducible to (K.C.1) and (K.C.2)? And how is this knowledge-how related to the subject's intention? To answer these questions, it is necessary to introduce the concept of affordance. DF's visuomotor actions are guided by affordances which are themselves constituted out of the relationship between properties of the subject of action (DF, in this case) and properties of the object of action (the postal slot) *and*, importantly, the subject's intention. The role of intention in shaping the affordance is an important part of what makes DF's retained visuomotor actions intelligent and therefore knowledge-based, rather than mere abilities.

4.4   The Role of Affordance in Intelligent Action

In a well cited passage, Gibson describes an affordance as that which is offered to the subject or animal (hereafter, subject): what it "provides or furnishes" whether "for good or ill" (Gibson 1979, 127). He also suggests that the affordance is independent of the subject; independent, that is, of his need and perception of it: "The affordance of something does *not change* as the need of the observer changes . . . The object offers what it does because it is what it is" (Gibson 1979, 139). Yet Gibson also states that "[d]ifferent layouts afford different behaviours for different animals" and, more explicitly, that an "affordance is relative to the size of the individual" (Gibson 1979, 128). A step, for example, will afford stepping onto or off relative to the size of the subject. A small subject-object ratio permits stepping, a large ratio may require the subject to jump or climb. Here, Gibson seems to be proposing that an affordance is neither strictly subjective nor strictly objective; instead, it is a relational property which provides information about both the environment and the subject (relative to each other). But how can this be if the affordance does not change and is determined by what the object is?

According to Natsoulas (2004), in order to disambiguate Gibson's descriptions of affordances, we must distinguish between an *affordance property* and *what an object affords*. Affordance properties, Natsoulas tells us, are invariant and offer what they do because of what the object is; but these are altogether different to what the object affords. (Natsoulas prefers the word 'independent' to 'invariant': for as he correctly points out, objects along with their properties may change over time, and therefore cease to be invariant, but they will always remain independent). What the object affords is constituted out of the *subject-object relation*. Thus, a stone has the independent affordance properties of graspability and throwability, but affords these only to a subject that can grasp and throw it. In relation to a mouse (for example), the affordance properties still exist, but they are not afforded the mouse.

With this distinction in place, it is now possible to make sense of Gibson's comments. Affordance properties, being properties of the object alone, are always there to be perceived (regardless of whether they are actually perceived), and are independent of the needs of the subject. On the other hand, what the object affords is relative to the subject and, as such, points neither to the subject nor the environment exclusively. What the object affords is a property that blurs the boundary between subjective and objective, just as Gibson declared. By adopting Natsoulas' distinction between the invariant (or independent) affordance properties, on the one hand, and the relational properties that an object affords, on the other, we can adopt a position that remains faithful to Gibson's description. Having made this distinction, however, from now on, when using the term 'affordance', I will be referring to what the object affords rather than its affordance properties.

If affordances (as I am using the term) constitute the relation between subject and object, then what exactly do we mean by subject? One suggestion is to define the subject in terms of body-scale (see Warren 1984, Warren and Whang 1987). In other words, the subject is defined in terms of his (or her) physical characteristics. However, according to Heft 1989, using body-scaling as a physical measure tells us little (or certainly not enough) about the subject's action capabilities. Yet it is these action capabilities, which are only *implied* by the physical description, that truly define the subject within the subject-object relation. This point is supported by Scarantino (2003) who describes how the graspability of an object relative to the physical measure of hand-span is inadequate in the case of a subject with an open but paralysed hand. Clearly, in this situation, the object is not graspable (by the subject), irrespective of any hand-span measurement we care to undertake. We could make the same point about the reachability of a book located on the top of a cabinet in relation to the height of a subject who is bedridden. With such examples in mind, Heft (1989) has developed what he considers to be a more fundamental and hence appropriate measure. Instead of body-scaling, Heft considered affordances to be relative to a subject's *potential for action*.[10] The significance of this more fundamental measure will become apparent in Section 4.5.

Having clarified what an affordance is, what does this have to do with the retained visuomotor capabilities of patient DF? Well, over the

---

[10]See Witt et al. (2005) for an interesting discussion on how intentional tool use affects the affordance of reachability.

years, a substantial amount of evidence has been amassed supporting the claim that humans (and other animals) possess two functionally distinct but complementary visual pathways (see Trevarthen 1968, Schneider 1969, Ungerleider and Mishkin 1982, Milner and Goodale 1995). Of particular interest, is a part of the visual system which divides into two extrageniculostriate projections. One—the ventral stream—projects to the inferotemporal cortex; the other—the dorsal stream—projects to the posterior parietal cortex. According to Milner and Goodale 1995, the ventral stream is implicated in the conscious perception and recognition of objects ('what the object is') whereas the dorsal stream is said to provide information for the visual guidance of skilled action (originally viewed as a 'where-the-object-is'-system, but now thought of as a 'how-to-engage-with-the-object'-system). In terms of immediate visuomotor action, it would seem that certain environmental demands are satisfied by the relatively crude discriminatory capacity inherent within the function of the dorsal stream (Goodale et al. 1986, Milner et al. 1991, Goodale and Milner 1992). Yet despite its importance for visuomotor action, evidence suggests that information processed along the dorsal stream makes little headway into consciousness.

For this and other reasons, Norman (2002) allies affordances with dorsal stream functioning.[11] As Norman correctly points out, Gibson claims that the pickup of affordances from within the optic array occurs without conscious awareness, or at least that consciousness is not necessary for the processing of affordances. Likewise, Gibson famously declares: "To perceive an affordance is not to classify an object" (Gibson 1979, 134). Again, we see a similarity with dorsal stream functioning, which does not involve the processing of representations and therefore the matching of them in memory for identification. In fact, evidence suggests that dorsal stream functioning occurs in the absence of representational[12] memory altogether (see Westwood and Goodale 2003, Goodale and Milner 2004). Through the functioning of the dorsal stream, an object is identified directly in action terms. As Gibson states: "You do not have to classify and label things in order to perceive what they afford" (Gibson 1979, 134); and again: "[T]he theory of information pickup does not need memory" (Gibson 1979, 254).

---

[11] According to Young (2006), a closer examination of the functioning of the dorsal stream, or rather the visuospatial capabilities of patients with certain visual pathologies related to its function, reveals problems with this strict alignment. Accumulated evidence from case studies involving other visual pathologies suggests that only *certain* affordances are processed along the dorsal stream. However, this debate need not impact on the discussion here, as Young (2006) argues that the affordances relevant to this discussion are processed via the dorsal stream.

[12] "Representational" does not necessarily entail conceptually articulable.

There are, it would seem, a number of similarities between the pickup of affordances and dorsal stream function. These are succinctly described by Schindler et al. (2004):

> When we reach out for an object, for example to pick up a cup, we use a set of exquisitely calibrated visuomotor processes in our brains that unthinkingly take into account the location and physical properties of the target object as well as the location and state of the body, arm and hand. Neurophysiological and functional MRI studies show that these brain systems are largely located around ... the so called 'dorsal stream'. (Schindler et al. 2004, 779)

Milner and Goodale (1995) hypothesised that DF's visual agnosia was caused by damage to the ventral stream of her visual system, resulting in a lack of object identification. However, her retained visuomotor skill is the result of an intact dorsal stream. This hypothesis has since been supported by fMRI scans taken of DF (see Culhan and Kanwisher 2001, James et al. 2003). DF is thus able to pickup affordances from within the optic array and process them via the dorsal stream as it projects to the posterior parietal cortex. Her retained visuomotor capability is therefore partly dependent on her being physically capable of moving her limbs in a way required to post the 'letter' through the slot; but this physical constitution also shapes the relational affordance. The postal slot affords 'post-slotability' because the slot allows the 'letter' to pass through it, and the subject has the physical constitution to pass the 'letter' through the slot. We have what Warren (1984) referred to as a *dynamic animal-environmental fit*. However, for an intelligent action to be a product of this 'fit', another important ingredient must be present—intention.

As noted earlier, knowing how to G consists in being able to G where G is an *intentional* act. Also noted earlier (when discussing beginner's luck), it is not enough simply to have the ability to G, or even to have successfully engaged in an act of G-ing; more than this, one must be *reliably* successful. One's reliable success must also match what one intended (recall Hawley), but the particulars of this intention need not be something that one is or can be consciously aware of. Nevertheless, because the particulars of one's intention help shape the nature of the affordance (thus making certain affordances available to the subject), and because the role played by these affordances is to elicit certain actions, the actions elicited by affordances are knowledge-based. In other words, it is not simply that DF has an ability to engage in action G (through performing p); rather, she intends to engage in action G; and this intention helps shape the affordance that guides the visuomotor activity (performance p). The cumulative effect of ability plus intention plus reliable success is a performance p that constitutes an intelligent action equivalent to (or that contributes to) knowing how to G. The fact that DF cannot articulate, or experience the particulars of performance p as she succeeds in G-ing means that she cannot satisfy (K.C.1) or (K.C.2). Consequently, what DF knows how to do cannot be reduced to any form of knowledge-that.

The role played by intention needs further clarification. DF intends to reach forward in an attempt to post the 'letter' through the slot. As such, she is not surprised when she reaches forward (because it is what she intended to do—or part of it at least). She is surprised specifically by her *success* at the postal-slot task. Her surprise is not because the particulars of her attempt are something she could not articulate (few of us probably could state the exact trajectory of the movement required to post the 'letter'); rather, it is because, unlike the vast majority of us, the particulars required for her success—the awareness of the slot's position and orientation in relation to oneself—are not something she is able to experience visually. Despite this, performance p (which amounts to more than just reaching forward) is intentional because its actualisation constitutes the act of G-ing (successfully posting the 'letter' through the slot). Achieving this goal—or at the very least, attempting to achieve it—constitutes the subject's *intentional project* (Young 2004).

The inter-related nature of performance p and the act of G-ing, where G is the intentional project—or superordinate goal—and p represents one or even a series of subordinate goals, can be found in non-pathological, even quite mundane, examples. To illustrate, suppose on one occasion my intentional project is to make a cup of tea (something that I have reflected on and therefore am aware of possessing). Within the framework of this superordinate goal (make a cup of tea), I proceed to fill the kettle with water, switch it on, place a teabag and sugar into a cup (etc.); all perhaps whilst listening to a broadcast on the radio, or even whilst talking to a friend on the telephone. Once I have engaged my intentional project, I will fill the kettle because it affords filling, and pick up a cup because it affords reaching for and grasping. Each subordinate action is itself intentional (despite the fact that it is not—certainly need not be—reflected on) because it is integrated within the (superordinate) intentional project of, in this case, making a cup of tea. Typically, we are aware of our intentional project; however, the particulars that contribute to the success of this overarching goal state inherit its intentionality without necessarily being something we are likewise aware of. The relationship between the subordinate and superordinate goal states is implied within one of the conditions of (CIA)—subject S

knows how to G if S is able to perform p (this can be a subordinate goal), rather than other than p, where p is a means (or even a part means) of intentionally G-ing.

The importance of affordance-based intelligent action is perhaps made all the more conspicuous when absent from the performance of the subject. To illustrate, consider the case of optic ataxia patient IG.

4.5 Patient IG: A Further Problem for Intellectualism

In contrast to DF, Milner et al. (2001) discuss the case of IG who, after suffering bilateral damage to the posterior parietal cortex, presents with a profound disorder of spatial orientation and visually guided reaching. Typically, IG is unable to grasp an object appropriately, even though she can identify the object and describe its location (in front of me, or to the right etc.). What is interesting about IG, particularly in contrast to DF, is that, despite profound deficits in real-time grasping, she is nevertheless able to demonstrate skilled pantomimed action (that is, grasping based on the visual recollection of an object in memory, rather than any current perception of it). By drawing on memory representations (acquired by previewing the object a few seconds earlier), IG is able to improve on her ineffective real-time grasping by employing a much more effective pantomimed grasp (see also Milner et al. 1999, 2003, Revol et al. 2003). Milner et al. (2001) conclude that IG's pantomime ability stems from some form of 'off-line' visuomotor guidance which operates independently of the dorsal stream projection to the posterior parietal cortex that guides the effective real-time grasping of DF.

Through the use of memory representations and pantomime grasping techniques, IG is able to retrieve an object presented in close proximity to her with reasonable ease. What is evident, then, is that IG possesses the physical ability to reach out and grasp the object—at least when using a memorised representation of its size and location to guide her. In other words, it is not that she simply cannot complete the task because of some global disruption to her hands and arms; rather, it is that she cannot retrieve the object using currently perceived information about its size and location. IG knows how to G (retrieve the object), in the sense proffered by intellectualism—namely, she knows that p is a way to G. She is also able to perform p and, in doing so, engage in the act of G-ing, but only under certain conditions or, conversely, only not under certain conditions. Of interest to the question of epistemic reduction pursued here, and my continuing challenge to intellectualism, are two inter-related questions: What is absent when IG fails to retrieve objects during *real-time* reaching and grasping? And, conversely, what is present to enable IG to retrieve objects during pantomimed tasks?

Is it that IG cannot directly retrieve the object because the affordances of reachability and graspability are not available to her? Earlier, we discussed how affordances are relational properties that constitute the potential for action between subject and object, and how this potential for action is in part based on the subject's physical capabilities. IG, we know, is physically capable of reaching for and grasping the object. As such, it seems reasonable to conjecture that these affordances should be available from within the optic array. Yet they do not elicit successful action, even when the subject intends to reach out and grasp the object. Perhaps, then, it is that the affordances are not *processed* appropriately owing to damage to the posterior parietal cortex. Might it be as Buxbaum and Coslett (1998) suggest: that optic ataxics are constrained by the wrong co-ordinates in their dysfunctional performance? Possibly: if we take 'wrong co-ordinates' to be the product of a disruption in the processing of affordances.

IG, in failing to retrieve the object in the real-time retrieval task, subsequently fails to demonstrate intelligent action. Yet, IG intends to retrieve the object (or at least try to), and she possesses the physical capability to carry this out. What she lacks, I conjecture, as with other optic ataxia patients, is the ability to process affordances. DF, in contrast, has retained this ability. Consequently, she is able to use the affordance to elicit appropriate intentional action, and in doing so demonstrate knowledge-how. The ability to process affordances is not knowledge-how; rather, it is the nature of the afforded property when actualised through a combination of intention and physical capability that constitutes knowledge-how. The nature of the affordance is, after all, shaped by—reciprocally determined, even—the physical capabilities and intentions of the subject, as well as the particular constitution of the object. As the subject's skill level increases, the nature of the affordance changes in accordance with this increase. The affordance is a measure of the subject's potential for action relative to the object: a potential which itself is a measure of the subject's skill. In other words, the nature of the affordance indicates the potential for intelligent action which, when actualised, constitutes knowledge-how to *G*. IG cannot actualise this potential for action because of her pathology. Consequently, she cannot demonstrate intelligent action (knowledge-how) when engaged in real-time retrieval.

So what changes for IG during the successful pantomime task, and is this change indicative of knowledge-how? We know that IG employs memory representations of the object when engaging in reaching and grasping. IG's retrieval behaviour is therefore mediated by mental imagery, rather than being elicited directly by affordances. According to Jung and Newen (2010), these images constitute a third type of knowledge which they describe as an "image-like knowledge format" (Jung and Newen 2010, 124). This form of knowledge cannot be captured by propositions, nor does it employ sensory information directly. Jung and Newen illustrate this 'third way' with an example of a ski jumper who uses image-like representations to improve his performance during training—the ski jumper can imagine a performance without engaging in the action. The image is more fined grained than propositions allow, insofar as the image is identified with an analogous code that retains the perceptual features and therefore detail of the object (Jung and Newen 2010); it also represents the action from the perspective of the agent without engaging affordances.

Does IG utilise Jung and Newen's image-like knowledge format? If knowing how to G in propositional terms (which IG does know) along with the physical capability to engage in performance p (which IG does have) were sufficient for G-ing, then presumably IG would be able to engage in real-time object retrieval. What IG is lacking, I have argued, is the ability to process affordances during the actualisation of real-time retrieval. It is this that prevents IG from knowing how to G, *qua* intelligent action. Could it be, then, that in pantomimed retrieval, where affordances are not available or even required, IG utilises an image-like knowledge format that is independent of knowing how to G (in propositional terms) that she already possesses, but is a necessary requirement, in conjunction with her physical constitution, for knowing how to G *qua* intelligent (pantomimed) action? This, of course, is an empirical question the answer to which is mere speculation at this stage. Nevertheless, IG does appear to be utilising knowledge-how that is more fine-grained than propositions (such as the object is in front of me, slightly to the right) when engaged in reaching and grasping: knowledge that is in keeping with Jung and Newen's image-like knowledge format, I suggest.

4.6   Conclusion

In concluding, it is important to note that it has not been my aim to present these case studies as the *only* demonstration of an irreducible species of knowledge-how. Certainly the case study approach is less orthodox than that taken by other contributors to the debate (however, see Adams 2009). What it does provide, I believe, is both the means for controlling and contrasting those variables implicated in the discussion on differences between knowledge-how and knowledge-that, and the opportunity to map these onto underlying neurological function and deficit. The double dissociation evident in the performances of DF and IG enable us to contrast the role of ventral and dorsal stream function, and affordances, in the pursuit of intelligent action; it has also allowed me a novel yet (I would say) informed way of arguing against intellectualism. DF, I have maintained throughout, satisfies (CIA) and, in doing so, demonstrates a species of knowledge-how that is resistant to reduction. In the case of IG, I have also speculated—albeit briefly—over the possible demonstration of another form of irreducible knowledge-how (the image-like knowledge format), although it may be that this can be reduced to knowledge-that. I wait further discussion on this issue, which the need for brevity does not permit here. Nevertheless, IG is an important example to include because of what she is *unable* to do. I have argued that the knowledge-how conspicuously absent from IG's real-time retrieval is the very thing which DF possesses. The culmination of affordance-based, reliably successful action satisfies (CIA) whilst systematically failing to meet the requirements of (K.C.1) and (K.C.2), and with it the intellectualist's reduction.

References

Adams, M.P. 2009. Empirical evidence and the knowledge-that/knowledge-how distinction. *Synthese* 170:97–114.

Ammerman, R. 1956. A note on 'knowing that'. *Analysis* 17 (2):30–32.

Bengson, J., M.A. Moffett, and J.C. Wright. 2009. The folk on knowing how. *Philosophical Studies* 142 (3).

Bermúdez, J.L. 2003. *Thinking without Words*. Oxford University Press.

Bermúdez, J.L. 2007. Thinking without words: An overview of animal ethics. *Journal of Ethics* 11:319–335.

Brown, D.G. 1971. Knowing how and knowing that, what. In O. Wood and G. Pitcher, eds., *Ryle*, pages 213–248. Macmillan.

Buxbaum, L.J. and H.B. Coslett. 1998. Spatio-motor representations in reaching: evidence for subtypes of optic ataxia. *Cognitive Neuropsychology* 15:279–312.

Carr, D. 1979. The logic of knowing how and ability. *Mind* 88 (351):394–409.

Carr, D. 1981. On mastering a skill. *Journal of Philosophy of Education* 15:87–96.

Culhan, J.C. and N.G. Kanwisher. 2001. Neuroimaging of cognitive functions in human parietal cortex. *Current Opinion in Neurobiology* 11:157–163.

Fantl, J. 2008. Knowing-how and knowing-that. *Philosophical Compass* 3 (3):451–470.

Gellner, G. 1951. Knowing how and validity. *Analysis* 12 (2):25–35.

Gibson, J.J. 1979. *The Ecological Approach to Visual Perception*. Houghton-Mifflin.

Gonzalez-Arnal, S. 2006. Non-articulable content and the realm of reasons. *Teorema* 25 (1):121–131.

Goodale, M.A. and A.D. Milner. 1992. Separate visual pathways for perception and action. *Trends in Neuroscience* 15:20–25.

Goodale, M.A. and A.D. Milner. 2004. *Sight Unseen: An Exploration of Conscious and Unconscious Vision*. Oxford University Press.

Goodale, M.A., A.D. Milner, L.S. Jakobson, and D.P. Carey. 1991. A neurological dissociation between perceiving objects and grasping them. *Nature* 349:154–156.

Goodale, M.A., D. Pelisson, and C. Prablanc. 1986. Large adjustments in visually guided reaching do not depend on vision of the hand or perception of target displacement. *Nature* 320:748–750.

Grego, J. 2009. Knowledge and success from ability. *Philosophical Studies* 142:17–26.

Grunbaum, T. 2008. The body in action. *Phenomenology and the Cognitive Sciences* 14 (2):243–261.

Hartland-Swann, J. 1956. The logical status of 'knowing that'. *Analysis* 16 (5):111–115.

Hawley, K. 2003. Success and knowledge how. *American Philosophical Quarterly* 40 (1):19–31.

Heft, H. 1989. Affordances and the body: An intentional anlysis of gibson's ecological approach to visual perception. *Journal for the Theory of Social Behaviour* 19 (1):1–30.

Hertherington, S. 2008. Knowing-that, knowing-how, knowing philosophy. *Grazer Philosophische Studien* 77:307–324.

Hornsby, J. and J. Stanley. 2005. Semantic knowledge and practical knowledge. *Proceedings of the Aristotelian Society – Supplementary Volume* 79 (1):107–130.

Hutto, D.D. 2005. Knowing what? Radical versus conservative enactivism. *Phenomenology and the Cognitive Sciences* 4:389–405.

James, T.W., G.K. Humphrey, A.D. Milner, and M.A. Goodale. 2003. Ventral occipital lesions impair object recognition but not object-directed grasping: an fmri study. *Brain* 126:2463–2475.

Johnson, M. 1991. Knowing through the body. *Philosophical Psychology* 4 (1):3–18.

Jung, E.-M. and A. Newen. 2010. Knowledge and abilities: The need for a new understanding of knowing how. *Phenomenology and the Cognitive Sciences* 9 (1):113–131.

Koethe, J. 2002. Stanley and Williamson on knowing how. *Journal of Philosophy* 99 (6):325–328.

Lihoreau, F. 2008. Knowledge-how and ability. *Grazer Philosophische Studien, Knowledge and Questions* Special issue:263–305.

McDowell, J. 1994. *Mind and World*. Harvard University Press.

McDowell, J. 1995. Knowledge and the internal. *Philosophy and Phenomenological Research* 55 (4):877–893.

Millikan, R.G. 2000. *On Clear and Confused Ideas: An Essay about Substance Concepts*. Cambridge University Press.

Milner, A.D., H.C. Dijkerman, R.D. McIntosh, Y. Rossetti, and L. Pisella. 2003. Delayed reaching and grasping in patients with optic ataxia. *Progress in Brain Research* 142:225–242.

Milner, A.D., H.C. Dijkerman, L. Pisella, R.D. McIntosh, C. Tilikete, A. Vighetto, and Y. Rossetti. 2001. Grasping the past: delay can improve visuomotor performance. *Current Biology* 11 (23):1896–1901.

Milner, A.D. and M.A. Goodale. 1995. *The Visual Brain in Action*. Oxford University Press.

Milner, A.D., Y. Paulignan, H.C. Dijkerman, F. Michel, and M. Jeannerod. 1999. A paradoxical improvement of misreaching in optic ataxia: New evidence for two separate neural systems for visual localization. *Proceedings of the Royal Society of London, B. Biological Sciences* 266:2225–2229.

Milner, A.D., D.I. Perrett, R.S. Johnston, P.J. Benson, T.R. Jordan, D.W. Heeley, D. Bettucci, F. Mortara, R. Mutani, E. Terazzi, and D.L.W. Davidson. 1991. Perception and action in visual form agnosia. *Brain* 114:405–428.

Moran, B.T. 2005. Knowing how and knowing that: artisans, bodies, and natural knowledge in scientific revolution. *Studies in History and Philosophy of Science* 36:577–585.

Natsoulas, T. 2004. "To See Is To Perceive What They Afford": James J. Gibson's Concept of Affordance. *Mind and Behaviour* 25 (4):323–348.

Noë, A. 2005. Against intellectualism. *Analysis* 65 (4):278–290.

Norman, J. 2002. Two visual systems and two theories of perception: An attempt to reconcile the constructivist and ecological approaches. *Behavioral and Brain Sciences* 25 (1):73–144.

Revol, P., Y. Rossetti, A. Vighetto, G. Rode, D. Boisson, and L. Pisella. 2003. Pointing errors in immediate and delayed conditions in unilateral optic ataxia. *Spatial Vision* 16:347–364.

Rosefeldt, T. 2004. Is knowing-how simply a case of knowing-that? *Philosophical Investigations* 27 (4):370–379.

Rumfitt, I. 2003. Savoir faire. *Journal of Philosophy* 100 (3):158–166.

Ryle, G. 1949. *The Concept of Mind*. Hutchinson.

Scarantino, A. 2003. Affordances explained. *Philosophy of Science* 70:949–961.

Schindler, I., N.J. Rice, R.D. McIntosh, Y. Rossetti, A. Vighetto, and D. Milner. 2004. Automatic avoidance of obstacles is a dorsal stream function: evidence from optic ataxia. *Nature Neuroscience* 7 (7):779–784.

Schneider, G.E. 1969. Two visual systems. *Science* 163:895–902.

Scott, W.T. 1971. Tacit knowing and the concept of mind. *The Philosophical Quarterly* 21 (82):22–35.

Sgaravatti, D. and E. Zardini. 2008. Knowing how to establish intellectualism. *Grazer Philosophische Studien* 77:217–261.

Snowdon, P. 2003. Knowing how and knowing that: A distinction reconsidered. *Proceedings of the Aristotelian Society* 105 (1):1–25.

Sosa, E. 2009. Knowing full well: The normativity of beliefs as performances. *Philosophical Studies* 142:5–15.

Stanley, J. and T. Williamson. 2001. Knowing how. *Journal of Philosophy* 98 (8):411–444.

Steel, T.J. 1974. A puzzle about knowing how. *Philosophical Studies* 25:43–50.

Toribio, J. 2008. How do we know how? *Philosophical Explorations* 11 (1):39–52.

Trevarthen, C.B. 1968. Two mechanisms of vision in primates. *Psychologische Forschung* 31:299–337.

Ungerleider, L.G. and M. Mishkin. 1982. Two cortical visual systems. In D. Ingle, M. Goodale, and R. Mansfield, eds., *Analysis of Visual Behaviour*, pages 549–586. MIT Press.

Upadhyaya, H.S. 1982. On knowing how and knowing that. *Indian Philosophical Quarterly* 9 (Supp):3–7.

Wallis, C. 2008. Consciousness, context, and know-how. *Synthese* 160 (1):123–153.

Warren, W.H. 1984. Perceiving affordances: Visual guidance in stair climbing. *Journal of Experimental Psychology: Human Perception and Performance* 10 (5):683–703.

Warren, W.H. and S. Whang. 1987. Visual guidance of walking through apertures: Body-scaled information for affordances. *Journal of Experimental Psychology: Human Perception and Performance* 13 (3):293–355.

Weiskrantz, L. 1986. *Blindsight*. Oxford University Press.

Weiskrantz, L. 1997. *Consciousness Lost and Found*. Oxford University Press.

Westwood, D.A. and M.A. Goodale. 2003. Peceptual illusion and the real-time control of action. *Spatial Vision* 16 (3/4):243–254.

Williams, J.N. 2008. Propositional knowledge and know-how. *Synthese* 165 (1):107–125.

Williamson, T. 2000. *Knowledge and its Limits*. Oxford University Press.

Winch, C. 2009. Ryle on knowing how and the possibility of vocational education. *Journal of Applied Philosophy* 26 (1):88–101.

Witt, J.K., D.R. Proffitt, and W. Epstein. 2005. Tool use affects perceived distance, but only when you intend to use it. *Journal of Experimental Psychology: Human Perception and Performance* 31 (5):880–888.

Young, G. 2004. Bodily knowing: Re-thinking our understanding of procedural knowledge. *Philosophical Explorations* 7 (1):37–54.

Young, G. 2006. Are different affordances subserved by different neural pathways? *Brain and Cognition* 62:134–142.

Young, G. 2009. Case study evidence for an irreducible form of knowing how to: An argument against a reductive epistemology. *Philosophia* 37 (2):341–360.

5

Understanding Knowledge in a New Framework: Against Intellectualism as a Semantic Analysis and an Analysis of the Mind

EVA-MARIA JUNG & ALBERT NEWEN

ABSTRACT

Since Stanley and Williamson (2001) rejected Ryle's well known dichotomy of knowing-how and knowing-that and argued for an intellectualist approach of knowing-how—i.e., for the thesis that knowing-how can be explained in terms of propositional knowledge—the persuasiveness of intellectualism has been revisited in various disciplines such as epistemology, philosophy of mind, psychology, and cognitive science. The aim of this paper is to show that two forms of intellectualism can be distinguished that are often admixed in recent debates. One kind of intellectualism is related to what can be called the "semantic project", the second one to the "knowledge representation project". We will argue that the first kind of intellectualism neglects the pragmatics of our language use whereas the second kind is not able to bridge the so-called "Knowledge-Action-Gap". Moreover, we will propose a new theoretical framework by distinguishing two forms of knowledge (practical and theoretical knowledge) and three knowledge formats (propositional, sensorimotor and image-like) that refer to different ways information constituting knowledge can be represented. We will try to show that our new framework allows for investigating the phenomenon of knowing-how as a common topic of philosophy and cognitive sciences.

Knowledge and Representation.
Albert Newen, Andreas Bartels
& Eva-Maria Jung (eds.).
Copyright © 2011, CSLI Publications.

5.1 The Rylean Approach to Knowing-how and Knowing-that

When Ryle introduced his seminal dichotomy of knowing-how and knowing-that (cf. Ryle 1945, 1949) he didn't know that his view would become focus on discussion during the turn of the 20th to the 21st century in philosophy, psychology and cognitive science. Ryle argues against a fictitious position he calls "intellectualist legend". According to that position, knowing-how can be explained through a chronologically ordered pair of activities: Firstly, a subject thinks of certain "regulative" propositions, rules or criteria for the planned actions; secondly, she puts into practice what these propositions purport. Ryle accuses the intellectualist legend of being caught in the grip of Cartesian Dualism that leads to a misconception of human intelligence. He presents the following two main arguments against this intellectualist approach:

1. It conflicts with the learning and applying situations of knowing-how we are familiar with in everyday life: Knowing rules or criteria for an action does not necessarily lead to successful practice, nor does learning how to do something always presuppose some theoretical knowledge of corresponding rules. Thus, there is a gap between knowing and acting that is left unexplained by the intellectualist (in the following, we will call this gap the "Knowledge-Action-Gap").

2. The intellectualist legend's conception of knowing-how leads to a vicious regress: Since thinking about a proposition is itself an action that can be done more or less intelligently, it corresponds to another knowing-how which, according to the legend, can be explained through a previous thinking about certain "regulative propositions", and so on.

In opposition to the intellectualist legend, Ryle argues for a strict dichotomy between knowing-how and knowing-that.[1] In his view, both have to be regarded as two different, irreducible manifestations of human intelligence: knowledge-that is theoretical knowledge of facts while knowledge-how consists in practical abilities, i.e., "multi-tracked dispositions" allowing a flexible, intelligent behavior acquired by training and experiences.

---

[1]In his 1945 paper, Ryle even goes further by arguing that the concept of knowledge-how is logically prior to the concept of knowledge-that (cf. Ryle 1945, 4). We will not discuss this argument since it is not relevant to the question we focus on in this paper.

We will not discuss whether Ryle's arguments against the intellectualist legend are persuasive[2] but let us remark that he was not arguing against an argumentatively strong position. In recent discussion, some authors present more sophisticated intellectualist positions, casting doubt on Ryle's positive characterization of knowing-how. Our aim is to show that this recent criticism discloses that Ryle's distinction is indeterminate since he mixes up two different projects connected to the question of the nature of knowing-how.

5.2 Ryle's Critics

In this section, we will consider the criticism against Ryle's identification of knowing-how with practical abilities. An array of putative counterexamples against this thesis has been developed recently. The first class of these examples is given in order to support the following thesis:

(i) Practical abilities are not *necessary* for knowing-how.

The argument runs like this: In various cases we ascribe knowledge-how to a subject even though she lacks the related ability. Snowdon argues that a cook still knows how to bake a cake even though he is hindered to perform his practical ability because the required sugar isn't handy (cf. Snowdon 2004, 8); Stanley and Williamson claim that a *maestra* who loses her arms in a bad accident (and, consequently, her practical ability to play the piano) can still be credited with the corresponding knowledge-how (cf. Stanley and Williamson 2001, 416). In the first example, the practical ability is hindered by *external circumstances*. Yet, this case doesn't present a persuasive argument against Ryle's position since having a practical ability doesn't imply that one is able to put it into practice wherever and whenever he wants to. Practical abilities are sensitive to environmental condition: I wouldn't lose my ability to ride a bicycle just because there is no bicycle handy.[3] The second example is more challenging: In this case, the practical performance is made impossible due to *internal, bodily conditions*. We can admit to Stanley and Williamson that the *maestra* won't lose all knowledge related to the practice of piano playing just because she is disabled to perform her ability. For reason that she is an expert in her field, we will expect that she is still able to explain how the actions can be well performed, or that she can teach others how to perform

---

[2]A more detailed discussion can be found in Stanley and Williamson (2001) and Noë (2005).

[3]Cf. also Noë (2005) who describes practical abilities as "embodied" and "situated".

them and judge whether performances are good or bad, etc. However, it is not clear whether these examples can successfully reject Ryle's thesis. Stanley and Williamson claim that the *maestra*'s knowing-how is independent of her actual ability. Yet, there's obviously a *reference problem*: Do we really mean the same when we ascribe knowing-how to the *maestra* before and after the accident? If we learn to play the piano and become experts after some time, our practical ability is usually attended by the acquirement of an array of different kinds of abilities and knowledge, for example, the ability to read music, the theoretical knowledge of different structures of piano pieces, or the ability to listen carefully to music performed by others. It is unclear whether accrediting the *maestra* with knowledge-how after the accident is just a way to acknowledge these pieces of knowledge and abilities she still possesses even though she has probably lost her knowledge how to play the piano (i.e., her practical skill). What Stanley and Williamson show by citing this example is that in our everyday language the reference of "knowing-how" is underdetermined: We can refer to the practical ability itself but also to another set of knowledge and abilities that is related to this ability. We will discuss this problem in more detail in Section 5.5.1. However, if we just accept that knowing-how, in one of its senses, refers to the practical ability, Ryle's account can successfully be defended against the putative counter-examples.

Another set of examples brought up against Ryle's view is given to support the following thesis:

(ii) Practical abilities are not *sufficient* for knowing-how.

White refers to abilities like hearing traffic, seeing across the room, holding five pints of beer, or doing without sleep for about 18 hours. He argues that all these abilities don't correspond with knowledge-how: we are *simply able* to perform them (cf. White 1982, 16). Snowdon cites the case of Martin who is able to perform fifty consecutive sit-ups arguing that Martin's ability is not related to a specific knowledge-how (cf. Snowdon 2004, 11). Regardless of how persuasive these objections are, Ryle could have answered them by specifying the concept of practical ability he identified with knowing-how. Thus, he could have excluded the cases White cites by considering only abilities sensitive to learning processes. Snowdon's case, in turn, discloses the need for an appropriate *individuation* of practical abilities. We do not ascribe a specific knowing-how to Martin since the ability to do *exactly fifty* consecutive sit-ups is, in general, not of interest. We would rather credit Martin with the ability to do sit ups (and the corresponding knowing-how, respectively) and emphasize that he is able to perform it with an impressive strength and endurance.

To conclude: The counter-examples show that Ryle's dichotomy needs some specification in order to cope with the reference problem of knowing-how and the under-determination of the concept of a practical ability. Therefore, a naïve identification of knowing-how with abilities might be too strong since the examples suggest that there is no strict synonymy between both concepts.

5.3   Stanley and Williamson's New Intellectualism

A possibility to reject Ryle's account is to argue for a persuasive analysis of knowing-how that successfully reduces it to knowing-that. This is the objective of Stanley and Williamson's (in the following: S&W) approach that has become the anchor-point of recent discussions. Knowing-how is, according to S&W, a species of knowledge-that, in the same way as other knowledge ascriptions like knowing where, who, why, etc, are kinds of propositional knowledge. In other words, if we ascribe the knowledge-how of, say, riding a bicycle to a subject, we indeed do ascribe knowledge-that to her. To support this claim, S&W analyze knowledge ascriptions in the light of contemporary theories of syntax and semantics. The analysis of their paradigmatic sentence "Hannah knows how to ride a bicycle" leads, according to them, to a "knowing-that"-clause since it is true

> [...] if and only if, for some contextually relevant way w which is a way for Hannah to ride a bicycle, Hannah knows that w is a way for her to ride a bicycle. (Stanley and Williamson 2001, 426)

S&W admit that this characterization of "knowing-how"-ascriptions is not complete. Since we can think of propositions in different ways, the analysis must be extended by clarifying which mode of presentation is connected to relevant instances of knowing-how. Therefore, S&W introduce a new kind of mode of presentation, a so-called "practical mode of presentation" (cf. Stanley and Williamson 2001, 429ff.), in order to do justice to the difference between a knowing how to ride a bicycle that we acquire only through, for example, observing other people riding bikes (and that, therefore, is represented in a demonstrative mode of presentation) and the relevant knowing-how going beyond this. S&W remark that this practical mode of presentation is related in "complex ways to dispositional states" (Stanley and Williamson 2001, 430). A detailed analysis is, according to them, only possible via reference to other modes of presentation: They claim that the use of it can be made intelligible through analogy to the "here"-mode of presentation introduced by Gareth Evans (cf. Evans 1982) and the "first-person"-mode of presentation referred to by John Perry (cf. Perry 1979, for further discussion see Newen 1997) in order to describe different functional roles of mental states within the discussion of indexicality.

We will discuss some problems confronting the "practical mode of presentation" in Section 5.5.1. At the moment our focus is on another question: Do S&W develop an analysis that can reject Ryle's analysis *in general*, i.e., are the conflicting analyses at all comparable? This question concerns the background assumptions and methodologies on which Ryle's and S&W's theories of knowing-how are based on. Let us explain this in more detail. Noë (2005) accuses S&W of deducing their explanation of "knowing-how" from recent linguistic theories about "knowing-how"-sentences. As he puts it:

> Ryle's distinction is not a thesis about the sentences used to attribute propositional and practical knowledge respectively. It is a thesis about the nature of practical and propositional knowledge. (Noë 2005, 287)

Stanley rejects this objection:

> Stanley and Williamson propose a thesis about the nature of knowing-how; they do not only make claims about sentences that ascribe knowledge-how. According to them, all of the reasons that have been given for rejecting propositional knowledge accounts of knowledge how can be accommodated by their view of its fundamental nature. (Stanley forthcoming, 14)

This leads to the following question: What *is* the nature of knowledge-how and what *methods* should we use in order to analyze it? In the following section we will show that Ryle's analysis leaves open this question and that at least two different projects can be identified based on two very different understandings of the nature of knowledge-how.

5.4   Ryle Revisited

On the one hand, Ryle's aim was to explain that our *ordinary notion* of knowing-how cannot be explained in terms of knowing-that: both notions belong, according to him, to different families of expressions. Whereas the former is connected to predicates like "intelligent", "clever", etc., the latter relates to those like "intellectual" or "well informed". Therefore, he seemed indeed to be aiming to provide a semantic analysis of knowledge-how. On the other hand, Ryle's aim was to show that there are two different ways of "exercising qualities of mind" (Ryle 1949, 25). In this way, Ryle's project goes beyond a semantic analysis of the concept of knowledge-how. It concerns the question of whether all mental cognitive processes can be analyzed in terms of propositional knowledge. Ryle's arguments against the intellectualist legend can be interpreted in this spirit: He accuses it of neglecting our everyday experiences concerning learning and applying knowing-how (and abilities, respectively). In other words, he argues that the intellectualist position is at conflict with the mental nature and the phenomenology of practical abilities. We will call the project related to this question the "knowledge representation" project since it concerns the question of how we gain and use information that constitutes knowing-how (in the sense of being able to act intelligently) and knowing-that, respectively.[4]

Now we see why Ryle's account is problematic: His approach to knowing-how and knowing-that crosses two different projects, namely, the "semantic analysis" project, on the one hand, and the "knowledge representation" project, on the other hand. Thus, his account affects both, questions in epistemology (mostly related to project 1) as well as questions in the philosophy of mind and the cognitive sciences (mostly related to project 2). The main aim of this paper is to argue that both projects should be kept apart since in the recent discussion of knowing-how and knowing-that many arguments are due to an illegitimate amalgamation of the two projects.

The same problem holds for the notion of intellectualism that is widely used in philosophy and cognitive science, yet not used consistently: the two different projects we characterized above correspond to at least two different intellectualist positions. Consider how Stanley describes intellectualism:

> Let us call *intellectualism* the view that knowing how to do something is a species of knowing that something is the case. (Chapter 3, 41)

S&W's intellectualism has to be understood in terms of the "semantic analysis" project: They vindicate intellectualism insofar as they hold that our ordinary notion of knowing-how can be exhaustively explained in terms of knowing-that. As Stanley puts it, the main objection to Ryle's account is that "[o]ur ordinary notion [of knowing-how] is not Rylean in character" (Stanley forthcoming, 2). Thus, the first kind of intellectualism can be defined in the following way:

Intellectualism₁ The phenomenon we refer to by using the concept of knowing-how can be defined through the phenomenon we refer to by using the concept of knowing-that.

---

[4]We do not want to argue for the claim that all questions about knowing-how can be covered by these two projects. There might be various other projects. What we aim to show, in the following, is that the recent debate on knowing-how and knowing-that is predominated by the merging of the two projects we named.

As we have already shown, the second project does not focus on our ordinary or folk-psychological notions of knowing-how and knowing-that but rather on the information processing systems underlying the phenomena usually associated with these notions. Therefore, the second kind of intellectualism can be defined in the following way:

Intellectualism₂ Information processes constituting knowing-how (and abilities, respectively)[5] can be reduced to information processes constituting knowing-that (factual knowledge).

In the following section we will discuss the two kinds of intellectualism in more detail.

5.5 Two Kinds of Intellectualism

5.5.1 Intellectualism₁: The "Semantic Analysis"-Project

Let us first consider intellectualism₁ and the "semantic analysis"-project, respectively. Intellectualism₁ is characterized by the thesis that our folk-psychological notion of knowing-how does not refer to a phenomenon irreducible to knowing-that, i.e., propositional knowledge, but can rather be explained in terms of it. This is to say that knowing-how denotes a relation between a subject and a proposition, and not (as Ryle suggests) between a subject and an ability (or anything else that is irreducible to propositional knowledge). We have shown that S&W accuse Ryle's analysis of not appropriately analyzing our everyday notion of knowing-how.

Ryle's "semantic analysis" project can be regarded as a follow-up project of the late Wittgenstein: Based upon the use of our ordinary concepts, he aims at presenting a philosophical account that can explain the mental phenomena (not only our speech of them). According to Ryle, our everyday concept of knowing-how is used in a way guided by an implicit understanding of the underlying phenomena. His aim is to reveal this understanding within a new theoretical framework. S&W's approach is quite different: They regard a paradigmatic sentence we use for ascribing knowledge-how and develop an appropriate linguistic analysis of this sentence based on recent theories of syntax and semantics. The key for supporting a reductive analysis of knowing-how lies, according to them, in the truth conditions of the sentence in question. From a linguistic perspective, S&W hold that (i) Ryle's analysis is wrong since it doesn't fit with the linguistic analysis, and (ii) "knowing-how"-sentences aren't ambiguous since the analysis leads

---

[5]Intellectualism within the second projects depends on how knowing-how is defined. Often, but not always, it is identified with practical abilities. See also Section 5.5.2.

unequivocally to an intellectualist claim. Of course, it is one of S&W's merits that they offer a systematic analysis including recent theories of syntax and semantics; Ryle's account misses these systematics and is more or less based on some linguistic intuitions. However, we argue that S&W do not offer a complete solution to the "semantic-analysis"-project.

In Section 5.2 we have shown that a naïve identification of knowledge-how with practical abilities (and of "knowing-how" with "can" or "being able", respectively) is obviously wrong. Thus, there is at least no synonymy between both concepts.[6] Other authors have already acknowledged this deficit in Ryle's account. As Edward Craig puts it: " 'Know how to' is indeed related to 'can', but not so closely as to justify synonymy" (Craig 1990, 155). For this reason, we introduced two different readings of "knowing-how"-sentences (cf. Jung and Newen 2010): a "propositional" reading, on the one hand, and an "ability" reading, on the other hand. This is in line with, for example, Jaakko Hintikka's distinction of the "knowing the way" sense and the "skill" sense of knowing-how:

> What is confusing about the locution 'knowing how' is that it has several different uses. On one hand, [...] "a knows how to do x" may mean that a has the skill and capacities required to do x, it may also mean that a knows the answer to the question: How should one go about it in order to do x? (Hintikka 1975, 11)

Thus, we are confronted with the following problem: Our folk-psychological notion of "knowing-how" does not refer to a single phenomenon. In this sense, Ryle's account seems to be compatible with Stanley and Williamson's since both do describe different senses of "knowing-how": the former the "ability", or "skill" sense, the latter the "propositional", or "knowing the way" sense. Yet, S&W are not convinced by this: They hold that the semantic analysis of "knowing-how"-ascriptions leads unequivocally to ascriptions of propositional knowledge (i.e., knowing-that) denying that the "ability" sense has any impact on the semantic project. In the following, we will argue that this is not a promising strategy.

The question is how the two senses of "knowing-how" are related to each other. Hintikka argues in the following way:

---

[6]However, we do not agree with Ryle's critics that he intended to defend this strong synonymy since he tried to specify what kinds of abilities are related to "knowing-how". According to Ryle only abilities that become manifest by "acquired, multi-tracked dispositions" (cf. Ryle 1949, 40ff.) count as knowledge-how. Thus, it is required that we can learn those abilities (vs. innate abilities) and that we have minimal control in exercising them (vs. mere habits).

> Of these, the skill sense seems to be largely parasitic on the other one. Its presence in ordinary discourse can be partly explained in terms of pragmatic (conversational) forces. (Hintikka 1975, 11)

This suggests that there is indeed no strict linguistic ambiguity of "knowing-how"-sentence. We can admit to S&W that the "propositional" sense has some priority over the "ability" sense. Moreover, it has many advantages to identify knowing-how as a species of knowing-that. Understood in this way it shows some core similarities to other kinds of propositional knowledge and can be related to traditional epistemic concepts like truth, belief, and justification. This allows for an integration of knowing-how into our traditional epistemological projects.[7] But can the "ability", or "skill" sense simply be neglected? As Hintikka puts it, it may at least count as an "unavoidable shadow of the 'knowing the way' sense." (Hintikka 1975, 12). A way to reject S&W would be to doubt that their semantic analysis is correct and that the skill-sense must indeed be included to it. In this line, Ian Rumfitt (2003) objects that S&W's linguistic argument doesn't succeed if it is formulated in several natural languages other than English. Stanley tries to respond to this objection by citing an array of paradigmatic cases from various languages (cf. Stanley forthcoming, sec. 5). Still, it is an open question whether S&W's account can be defended against this cross-linguistic argument. However, S&W's view seems to be supported by recent studies in experimental philosophy: Bengson et al. (2009) have provided a series of studies in which people were presented by several stories corresponding to the examples brought up in the debate and had to judge whether the subjects in question are able to perform an action, or know how to perform an action. They conclude that the folk-psychological notion of knowing-how is intellectualist rather than Rylean and doesn't show any ambiguity. Yet, it is difficult to interpret the results of those empirical studies: The situations described in those experiments are quite artificial. The participants were not free to judge the situations by their own words, but rather had to do a multiple-choice test that already suggested a difference in meaning of "knowing-how" and "ability". Therefore, the studies cannot be treated as strong evidence for intellectualism$_1$.

Our aim is to criticize S&W's account from a different point of view: We claim that their analysis of knowing-how does itself include pragmatics and therefore doubts the basis for neglecting the pragmatic

---

[7]Some authors have argued, however, that knowing-how understood in S&W's way differs from other forms of propositional knowledge. Poston (2009), e.g., doubts that it can be subject to Gettier-cases. We will not focus on this discussion here since our argument doesn't rely on this.

"skill" sense of the semantic analysis project. Let us explain this in more detail.

S&W's approach is confronted with a severe problem: Since they do not specify how a "practical mode of presentation" can be understood, it remains dubious whether they *de facto* present an argument for a complete reduction of knowing-how to knowing-that. Stanley tries to specify what is meant by "entertaining a practical mode of presentation" by saying:

> I only think of a way of doing something under a practical mode of presentation if I am disposed to employ it under various counterfactual circumstances. I may think of the very same way under a demonstrative mode of presentation, without having such dispositions. Of course, it is no easier to say what these dispositions are in the case of practical modes of presentation than in the case of "here" thought or "I" thoughts. But it is also no harder. (Stanley forthcoming, 6)

However, in case of spatial and indexical knowledge, the "here"- and the "first-person"-mode of presentation are related to certain *objects* (places and persons) whereas the practical mode of presentation is used to describe different *relations to facts*. Yet, it is unclear how these facts, in the case of practical abilities, can be individuated: It is hard to identify the propositions Hannah should know in order to be credited with relevant knowing-how. S&W presuppose that our knowledge how to ride a bicycle refers to the same ways of acting in case of merely regarding a person riding a bike (demonstrative mode of presentation) and in the more practical sense of "real" knowing-how (practical mode of presentation). And exactly this presupposition is questionable. As Jennifer Hornsby puts it:

> The problem is that the account requires identities between demonstrable ways of ϕ-ing (on the one hand) and such ways of ϕ-ing as go hand in hand with knowing how to ϕ (on the other hand); and there are not such identities. (Hornsby 2007, 179)

The problem lies in the facts or propositions that S&W assume to constitute cases of knowing-how. Stanley denies that propositional knowledge is bound to the verbal ability to express the constituents of the proposition grasped, *a fortiori* the proposition itself. As an example for a case of "grasping a proposition" not meeting this condition of verbal expressibility he cites the following case:

> The 8 year old Mozart can assert the proposition that constitutes his knowledge how to compose a symphony; he can just say, while composing it, the German translation of "this is how I can do it". (Stanley forthcoming, 8)

What can be deduced from this example? If we do ascribe propositional knowledge to little Mozart, our analysis of knowledge-how includes pragmatics in the sense of practical application and ability. And this indeed is what S&W want to avoid. Thus, the problem with S&W's analysis lies in the transformation of "knowing-how"-sentences to "knowing the way"-sentences: the knowing-how S&W analyze indeed differs from other propositional knowledge for which the object of knowledge can easily be identified. Even though, as S&W suggest, the possession of knowing-how enables Mozart to answer a question, his answer differs from the answer he would give if we ask him, for example, "What is the capital of France?". Thus, a deeper understanding of what is involved in the "propositional", or "knowing the way" sense may involve some degrees of pragmatism and, therefore, undermines S&W's strategy.[8]

To sum up: Referring to ways for acting under a practical mode of presentation seems to be incompatible with a purely semantic analysis of knowing-how utterances as long as the practical mode of presentation is characterized by dispositions. Since S&W's account of a practical mode of presentation is essentially relying on pragmatic considerations including an introduction of dispositions, there does not remain any convincing argument for neglecting the "ability", or "skill"-sense of knowing-how. In Section 5.6 we will suggest that the "semantic analysis"-project leads us to two different notions of knowledge even though these notions do not parallel the notions of knowing-how and knowing-that: We have seen that the former notion cannot be characterized fruitfully by a single analysis since two senses are applicable to it.

5.5.2   Intellectualism₂: The "Knowledge Representation"-Project

The core question of the second project is: How does the mind work? How do we represent knowledge? Many empirical sciences are concerned with this question. So, there's no wonder why Ryle's dichotomy of knowing-how and knowing-that has been used for a long time in cognitive sciences, philosophy of mind, psychology, and neurosciences. It goes along with several other dichotomies as procedural and declarative knowledge and memory, explicit and implicit knowledge and memory as well as implicit and explicit learning. Yet, these notions are neither strongly parallel nor defined uniquely in the literature.[9] Thus, if we are concerned with the second project, we have to be careful to judge

---

[8]For a similar objection against S&W see Stout (2010).

[9]For an overview of the various definitions see Eysenck et al. (1994), especially page 93, and Anderson (1980).

intellectualist positions: It is often not clear which distinction is indeed rejected. We will not discuss this problem in detail.

For the sake of argument, we only want to emphasize one point: Some authors (cf. Adams 2009) suggest that S&W's approach can be refuted since the differentiation of two different information processing systems in the brain is empirically grounded. However, we have seen that this is not a legitimate argument against S&W's theory since it crisscrosses the two different projects that are orthogonal to each other. In the following, we will focus on intellectualism$_2$ more directly by discussing two seminal positions: Fodor's (1968) account and the more recent theory of Dienes and Perner (1999).

In his 1968 article *The Appeal to Tacit Knowledge in Psychological Explanation* Fodor focuses on the paradigmatic example of the ability to tie one's shoes. His starting point is a homunculi explanation of the functions underlying this capacity: One should imagine that a little man lives in the head keeping a library that entails a volume on the method of "tying one's shoes". The little man presses buttons that activate mechanisms implying behavioral patterns. This model is intellectualist because it describes a way in which the performance of successful action can be reduced to the knowledge of rules guiding the successful action of shoe-binding. Fodor tries to defend such "intellectualist accounts of mental competences" (Fodor 1968, 627). He regards some objections that can be made against those models and tries to reject them:

(1) The objection that the model doesn't explain the details adequately concerns, according to Fodor, an empirical question and can't be seen as an objection to the model *in general*: If the detailed and complex mechanisms of tying one's shoes are known, then it remains the questions of whether the model gives an adequate description of the representations in mind when tying one's shoes. The question is, therefore, whether the model is *methodologically* wrong.

(2) The objection that the model leads to a vicious regress on the bases that the little man always has to know how to apply the rules he regards as important for the successful performance can also be rejected: There are things that we can simply do, i.e., *elementary operations* not depending on rules. These operations avoid the threatened regress.

(3) The objection that the model is inadequate because we usually cannot explain the rules underlying our intelligent actions like tying our shoes is rejected by Fodor through reference to the existence of "tacit knowledge", a technical term used in psychology. This notion plays a central role for his reductive analysis of the performance of abilities to propositional knowledge. As he puts it:

The problem can be put in the following way. Intellectualists want to argue that cases of X-ing involve employing rules, the explication of which is tantamount to a specification of how to X. However, they want to deny that anyone who employs such rules, *ipso facto*, knows the answer to the question "How does one X?" What, then, *are* we to say is the epistemic relation an agent necessarily bears to rules he regularly employs in the integration of behavior? There is a classical intellectualist suggestion: If an agent regularly employs rules in the integration of behavior, then if the agent is unable to report these rules, then it is necessarily true that the agent has *tacit* knowledge of them. (Fodor 1968, 636)

And later on:

Now I want to say: If X is something an organism knows how to do but is unable to explain how to do, and if S is some sequence of operations, the specification of which would constitute an answer to the question "How do you X?", and if an optimal simulation of the behavior of the organism X-s by running through the sequence of operations specified by S, then the organism *tacitly knows* the answer to the question "How do you X?" and S is a formulation of the organism's tacit knowledge. (Fodor 1968, 638)

The line of argument is quite clear: Through an inference from the operations underlying a successful simulation of our behavior Fodor holds that our ability to tie our shoes can be reduced to propositional knowledge even though the knowledge of the operation remains tacitly (implicitly) represented.

However, Fodor's approach is problematic for two main reasons: Firstly, his inference from processes underlying a machine's performance to the processes of the mind is not justified. Why should the mind work in exactly the same way as the simulator only because it leads to the same behavioral output? And secondly, his account does not explain the "Knowledge-Action-Gap" Ryle was hinting at. The assumption of "tacit knowledge" seems to be an *ad-hoc* hypothesis rather than an appropriate explanation of the ongoing processes that guide our intelligent behavior.

Another more recent intellectualist theory of knowledge-how is presented by Zoltan Dienes and Josef Perner (1999) (in the following: D&P). They develop a fine grained representational theory of knowledge according to which the two forms of knowledge can best be explained through implicitly and explicitly represented aspects of propositional knowledge. D&P suggest the source for implicitness lies in the fact that the information conveyed implicitly concerns supporting facts that are necessary for the explicit part to have the meaning it has. They define implicit and explicit representations in the following way:

> In our analysis the distinction is between which parts of the knowledge are explicitly represented and which parts are implicit in either the functional role or the conceptual structure of the explicit representations. A fact is explicitly represented if there is an expression (mental or otherwise) whose meaning is just that fact; in other words, if there is an internal state whose function is to indicate that fact. Supporting facts that are not explicitly represented but must hold for the explicitly known fact to be known are *implicitly represented*. (Dienes and Perner 1999, 736)

Thus, D&P's analysis is based on Fodor's Representational Theory of the Mind (in the following: RTM). They suggest that we should think of knowledge as a propositional attitude. According to this theory representations like "This is a cat" constitute knowledge if they are stored in a so-called "knowledge-box". Thus, their functional role lies in a reflection of a state of the world (in comparison to desired states that are thought of to be stored in a "goal box"). D&P first regard a coarse-grained distinction between self (holder of the attitude), the attitude ("knowing") and the content ("what is known"). They go on with more fine-grained distinctions concerning these parts in order to develop a hierarchical model allowing for a scale of more or less explicitly represented knowledge. Their paradigm case is visually guided knowledge, namely the perceptual knowledge of a cat sitting in front of the knowing subject. At the first end of the scale there is knowledge were only one part of the content, namely the property (e.g., "being a cat") is explicitly represented whereas all the other components remain implicit. This is the case when subjects are only able to name a presented object ("cat") but do not explicitly know any other part of the knowledge-relational components. At the other end of the scale is "fully" explicit knowledge that is marked through an explicit representation of all the parts they describe. In this case, not only does the subject fully and explicitly represent all parts of the content known but also has explicit knowledge about her attitude (knowing) and is aware of herself as the holder of this attitude.

However, also D&P's account is confronted with several problems. Ingar Brinck (1999), for example, objects that the model may describe visually guided knowledge adequately, but that it doesn't allow for an explanation of *practical competences*. Those competences are usually based on what is called "nonconceptual representations" that cannot be described as constitutents of propositional beliefs. Moreover, those nonconceptual representations are related to "correctness conditions" rather than to "truth condition" as D&P suggest (cf. Brinck 1999, 760–1). The authors answer to this objection by claiming that all characteristics that are usually ascribed to nonconceptual representations can be ascribed to the partially known content in case of implicit knowledge within their model (cf. Dienes and Perner 1999, 792). This might be true. In this case, however, the model D&P present doesn't seem to be a clear intellectualist model of knowledge representation any more. Rather, it tries to integrate anti-intellectualist tendencies. But this seems to be very misleading: Since they use RTM as a background assumption for their account (and this theory is, by definition, an intellectualist theory), they seem to present an anti-intellectualist model that is captured by intellectualist termini. Let us explain this a little bit more in detail: The suggestion that all the forms of implicit and explicit knowledge D&P describe can be explained on the basis of RTM suggests that these forms of knowledge are based on the very same representational format. And this assumption is usually seen as the core question in the conflict between anti-intellectualists and intellectualists. Holding that their theory allows for other representational formats (nonconceptual contents), too, undermines the strategy they use: why should we characterize nonconceptual representations as implicit conceptual components? In this case, RTM seems just to be a background theory that presupposes only one structure of knowledge (a propositional structure) but remains explanatory unfruitful and misleading. It is only a way to ascribe all forms of knowledge from an outside-perspective and judges what components remain implicitly represented by classifying the behavior of the subject in question. It remains unexplained how the implicit components are connected with our practical abilities. Therefore, D&P are also not able to bridge the "Knowledge-Action-Gap".

To conclude: Neither Fodor's description of practical knowledge based on the Language of Thought-Hypothesis nor D&P's more fine-grained theory relying on RTM offer a fruitful analysis since they fail in bridging the "Knowledge-Action-Gap". Thus, intellectualism$_2$ loses its attraction: The need for other representational formats than language-like representations becomes obvious. In Section 5.7 we will present a threefold approach to knowledge formats that avoids some of the problems intellectualist theories are confronted with.

5.6 Two Notions of Knowledge

In this section, we will focus on the semantic analysis project and develop a dichotomy of theoretical and practical knowledge that catches some of Ryle's core intuitions although not conforming to his approach.

We suggest differing between theoretical and practical knowledge in the following way: Theoretical knowledge, the most important form of knowledge in epistemology, describes a relation between a subject and a proposition thereby being related to a *norm of truth*. It is a focus of the "justified-true-belief"-analysis and of traditional epistemological questions, for example, the question what does count as reliable justification of our beliefs to be classified as knowledge. Practical knowledge, instead, describes a relation between a subject and an activity. This knowledge is related to the norm of success: We ascribe some ability to a person if she is able to successfully perform it.

Note that the two notions of knowledge essentially differ: Whereas the notion of theoretical knowledge denotes a "mind-to-world" direction of fit, the notion of practical knowledge is related to a "world-to-mind" direction of fit. Moreover, it is misleading to identify an object of knowledge in the case of practical knowledge: There simply is not such an object since it denotes a very different structure. It doesn't refer to an adequate thinking or believing about the world, but rather to successfully performed intentional actions.

Beyond these differences, there are also many similarities between the two notions: We have seen that the naïve identification of practical knowledge with abilities doesn't account for our intuitions. In most of the cases, we demand more than successful action; we expect the subject to perform the action in question in various circumstances. Katherine Hawley (2003) has addressed this problem by proposing an account of "knowing-how" (in our terms: of practical knowledge) as successful action plus warrant. To specify how this warrant is understood she offers a counterfactual analysis that is similar to Robert Nozick's (1981) counterfactual analysis of theoretical knowledge. A similar claim is made by Peter Markie (2006) who emphasizes the need for a justification or reliability of practical knowledge:

> To know how to engage in an activity is to internalize some norms directing the performance of particular ways of acting in various circumstances in order to engage in the activity, where those ways of acting in those circumstances are, in fact, reliable ways of engaging in the activity. (Markie 2006, 22)

Another problem concerning the analysis of practical knowledge concerns the activities that are correlated with practical knowledge. We do not assume that the performance of each and any activity counts as practical knowledge, but rather demand that the activities have to be performed intentionally and can be minimally controlled by the subject. Patricia Hanna (2006) addresses this problem and distinguishes between random or non-purposive activities that do not correspond to any knowledge, skills which we know how to perform, and "reasoned skills" for which rules play a special role. Those skills are, according to her, only successfully performable in case we consciously know the corresponding rules, i.e., in case we indeed have theoretical knowledge about them.

To avoid any misunderstandings: Our aim is not only to criticize intellectualism about knowing-how and knowing-that, but also to provide a new starting point for tackling the problem Ryle had in mind. We think that defining practical and theoretical knowledge in the way we suggest offers an alternative to the mere confrontation of intellectualism and anti-intellectualism.

5.7 Knowledge Formats – a Threefold Approach

In this section, we will focus on the second project—the knowledge representation project. We have seen that intellectualism$_2$ is not convincing since it doesn't do justice to our questions concerning how we extract and represent information from the environment that enable us to successfully perform actions. We propose a threefold analysis distinguishing (1) a propositional knowledge format, (2) a nonconceptual sensorimotor knowledge format, and (3) an image-like knowledge format. We try to support our threefold theory of knowledge formats by arguing for specific representations that are systematically distinguishable: (i) propositional representations, (ii) sensorimotor representations and (iii) image-like representations. We start with an unproblematic characterization of propositional representations. In a second step we illustrate all three kinds of representations presenting paradigmatic examples and argue that those representations are mutually different.

Propositional representations can be identified with linguistic or language-like representations (see, for example, Peacocke 1992). A mental representation is propositional if and only if the representation has an internal structure like a natural language. This involves the central features of a natural language (cf. Fodor 1998) including compositionality, systematicity, productivity, a strong stimulus independence as well as inferential relations. There is broad consensus that propositional representations have to be characterized in that way.

However, during the last decades the assumptions that all representations are structured by the Language of Thought has become under attack. The insight that there is intelligent behavior that can't be explained as being based on propositional representations has led to the assumption of nonconceptual representations.[10] Even though those representations allow for a minimal flexible behavior they are essentially stimuli dependent. The differentiation between propositional and nonconceptual, sensorimotor representations in humans has been demonstrated for visual knowledge on the basis of Milner and Goodale's (1993) so-called two visual system hypothesis.[11]

Also in representations of actions which are the main focus of our paper the role of nonconceptual content has been emphasized recently. Jeannerod (1997), for example, assumes that our actions are initiated by nonconceptually, "pragmatically" represented goals of action. Moreover, the guidance of our actions relies on sensorimotor representations that have as their content the movements of our body from the starting to the intended state and allow for smooth and precise executions. In general, sensorimotor representations include the information that is provided by what Gibson (1979) called "affordances", i.e., qualities of the environment that allow subjects to perform certain actions. Affordances ascribe a close relationship between perceptions and actions: By perceiving the affordance properties of graspability and drinkability a subject might reach out for the glass of water when she is thirsty.[12] Since sensorimotor representations are usually unconscious they enable us to smoothly interact with the environment in order to achieve our ends.

We think that to emphasize the role of nonconceptual representations for action is a good starting point to bridge the "Knowledge-Action-Gap". However, the distinction between propositional and nonconceptual representations is too coarse-grained to capture all cognitive processes bound to our abilities. Therefore, it is necessary to introduce a third representational format: *image-like* representations. This assumption is mirrored by Jeannerod's (1997) notion of "motor images" that describe a conscious access to usually unconsciously represented motor-patterns.

How can we characterize image-like representations in more detail? In basic actions like walking, grasping an object etc. we seem to rely simply on basic sensorimotor representations which are only activated if we receive an actual perceptual input as key stimulus. The key stimulus, for example, seeing a glass of water, may be the stimulus to grasp it given the situation of being thirsty. Sensorimotor representations differ

---

[10]See, for example, the discussion of the homing behavior of ants that supports the explanatory force of nonconceptual representations (Müller and Wehner 1988, Gunther 2003, Newen and Bartels 2007).

[11]See, for example, Young's discussion of patient DF in Chapter 4 of this volume.

[12]For a more detailed discussion of affordances see Chapter 4 of this volume.

from the image-like representations which we need to realize complex motor skills. Before presenting some examples let us highlight the distinguishing features: The claim is that we have to presuppose image-like representations (1) that are systematically connected with perceptual images and sensorimotor representations (as opposed to linguistic symbols which can be completely independent from any imagination), (2) that can nevertheless be activated independent from key-stimuli, for example, we can activate these representations by imagination (not only by actual perception), (3) that are forming an analog pattern, (4) that can be connected with other image-like patterns (connectability). Criterion 4 accounts for two cases: (a) image-like representations can be connected with sensorimotor representations, to perform an intended action which the subject wasn't able to perform without this new representational unity (see discussion of rotation ability below), (b) image-like representations can be connected with other image-like representations to form a new complex image, i.e., that allows the subject to imagine an action she never has performed before (see discussion of the tennis-example below).

There are several phenomena we can only account for if we presuppose image-like representations that are, on the one hand, non-propositional but, on the other hand, clearly different from basic non-conceptual sensorimotor representations depending on actual perceptual inputs. In a study of motor skills, Franz Mechsner et al. (2001) asked participants to rotate with both hands on a special apparatus (see Figure 1 on the facing page). If being asked to rotate with both hands in a parallel synchronous circling pattern (0 degree difference) or in an antiphase pattern (180 degree difference), they could easily realize the tasks by relying on image-like representations of the intended rotation-schema. Mechsner introduced two flags on top of each side of the rotation equipment that allow us to visually control the parallel or the antiphase rotation.

If being asked to rotate both hands such that one performs four circles with the left hand while one has to perform only three circles with the right hand at the same time, the participants were not able to do that. They simply did not have the image-like representation required. Mechsner then connected the flags above the left crank with the flag above the right hand (due to a gear system) such that, if the participants performed the 4 to 3 rotation with their hands, then the flags were rotating with the same frequency. In this case they could activate the image-like representation of such isofrequent flags again (which was already used before) and quickly learned to rotate in a 4 to 3 relation which had been impossible without this change of equipment.

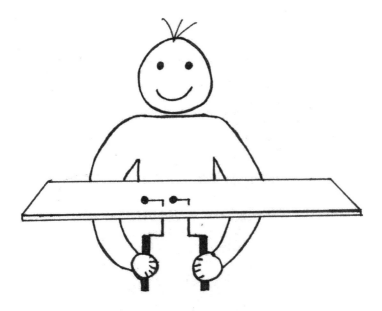

FIGURE 1 Experimental set-up of motor-skill study
by Mechsner et al. (2001).

The important lesson here is that we need an image of the rotation schema to realize the complex movement.

A second study supports the claim that the representations which allow us to realize complex motor behavior actually fulfill the criteria of image-like representations. One activity which is carefully studied is playing tennis (Schack and Mechsner 2006). The authors argue that complex motor activities like playing tennis are essentially relying on a special type of perceptual-cognitive representation which they call basic action concepts (BACs).[13] Basic action concepts like throwing a ball, bending the knee, bending the elbow, turning one's body, racket acceleration, stretching the whole body, etc. (11 BACs are identified with tennis) are organized and stored in memory as perceptual events (cf. Schack and Mechsner 2006, 77). This immediately shows that the

---

[13]According to our understanding these representations remain nonconceptual because they are not interdependent in a minimal holistic network although they are used to build connections (minimal connectability). The role of minimal holism as a necessary condition for a theory of concept possession is developed and defended in Newen and Bartels (2007). For the discussion here is sufficient to show that these representations are nonpropositional on the one hand but nevertheless distinguishable from basic sensorimotor representations.

first two criteria for image-like representations are satisfied: These representations are connected with images and are independent from actual perceptual inputs because they are stored in long-term memory and can be activated in quite different situations. Let us have a look at criteria 3 and 4: Given that, typically, we have pictorial representations these representations remain analog although they reach some level of abstractness. The information is analog because it contains a lot of gradually represented information, for example the velocity and direction of throwing the ball is not represented in a digital format. A digital representation focuses on one feature of an entity (including processes) and classifies that feature into one clear subcategory of several subcategories relative to one dimension (for example, the ball was hit soft, medium or hard). The image-like representations remain analog by relying on the gradual representation of the force, velocity etc. Finally, these basic action concepts can be connected to represent an integrated, more complex behavior, for example, 11 BACs form the units that can be combined to represent an activity like hitting a serve or returning a ball using a backhand grip. The connectability of BACs differs from the compositionality and systematicity of linguistic concepts. BACs only allow for extremely constraint connections and remain dependent on the activation of the relevant images. The characteristic independence of linguistic symbols from any kind of perceptual input and perceptual images is not realized on this level. On the other hand, the level of abstractness is already independent from actual perceptual inputs; that is the characteristic feature of basic sensorimotor representations.[14] Therefore, the representations involved in playing tennis are image-like representations which constitute a third independent level of representational format for abilities.

Image-like representations allow for mental training which is an important part of preparation in high-level sports performances. And it now becomes clear why this is possible. The image-like representations

---

[14]We do nor claim that sensorimotor representations aren't connected with perceptions at all; they are basically connected with situation-dependent actual perceptual inputs while image-like representations are essentially constituted by memory-based representations of images (in one of the sensory modalities) which can be activated independently from a key-stimulus and from any specific actual perceptual input. Furthermore, the study of Schack and Mechsner (2006) shows that experts usually develop a fine-grained cognitive structure of BACs with an hierarchical organization that fits the functional structure of the ability of playing tennis. The non-players had a comparably poor structure and their representations remained much more situation-dependent. Although Schack and Mechsner tend to speak only of one representational format of actions, we think that the strong differences between non-players and players supports our theoretical perspective. They simply ignore the important aspect of situation-dependence versus -independence.

are connected with mental images. They can be activated independently from an actual performance situation such that a sports person can start optimizing the mental representations that guide the performance. Let us switch to some support from the area of music: It is shown by Zatorre et al. (1996), Zatorre and Halpern (2005) that in cases of imaging music we can observe an activation of the auditory cortex that is very similar to the activation in the situation of actual listening to music. Furthermore, in the 2005 article the authors report from mental training of musical instruments and the effect that the musicians can "hear" their instrument during these mental trainings. There are further effects of musical imagination described by Sacks (2007): Beethoven was only able to continue composing after suffering from complete deafness because he has developed a very intense musical imagination which we would characterize as a paradigmatic case of image-like representations (Sacks 2007, ch. 4). Image-like representations seem also to be the relevant basis for phantom imaginations in the case of lost body parts: The well-known case of Paul Wittgenstein (a brother of famous Ludwig), a pianist who lost his right arm during the First World War, mirrors this. Wittgenstein was nevertheless able to imagine how to perform a new piece with his right hand long after the accident happened. He developed image-like representations allowing him to work out perfectly the relevant *Fingersatz* for the right hand (Sacks 2007, ch. 21).[15]

To summarize these evidences: It seems necessary to presuppose image-like representations which are still analog but independent from actual sensory inputs while not fulfilling the criteria of propositional representations (systematicity, productivity, compositionality). Especially mental training is presupposing these image-like representations.

5.8   The Specification of Action

In this section, we will show how Pacherie's (2008) recent approach to the phenomenology of action conforms with our threefold analysis of knowledge formats. We take this to be an additional support for our new framework since practical knowledge and the nature and phenomenology of intentional actions are closely interconnected. Pacherie develops a new conceptual framework allowing for a more precise characterization of the many facets of the phenomenology of action by expanding the two-fold theories suggested by, for example, Searle's (1983) distinction between prior intentions and intentions-in-action, and Mele's

---

[15]Note that phantom imagination differs from mere phantom pain since they are related to images of actions once performed with the phantom limb.

(1992) distinction between distal and proximal intentions, into a three-fold theory of intentions. She argues for a distinction between three main stages in the process of action specification, each corresponding to a different level of intention (i.e., distal, proximal, and motor intentions) and each level of intention having a distinctive role to play in the guidance and monitoring of the action.

According to Pacherie, the first step of action specification can be characterized by distal intentions (D-intentions) their main function is the rational guidance of our actions, i.e., they terminate practical reasoning about the aim of our action and about the appropriate means and plans to achieve this aim, and they coordinate intra- and interpersonal levels. Since the content of those intentions is conceptual and at least partly describable we can relate it to our network of intentions, beliefs, and desires. Although not completely context-free the forming of D-intentions doesn't strongly depend on the particular situations of the agents. However, this means that the initial description of the intended type of action is very coarse-grained and leaves indeterminate many aspects of the action by not including all the aspects of the situation at hand.

The second step can be characterized through proximal intentions (P-intentions) which are concerned with the generation of an intention to start acting at a given time and situation. Their main function is to anchor our rational action plan in the particular situation of action. Pacherie claims that P-intentions involve an integration of perceptual and conceptual information, i.e., the agent must generate an indexical representation of the action to be performed and be sure that the implementation of the action conforms to the rationally chosen action plan.

Finally, the third step is characterized by motor intentions (M-intentions) that are responsible for the precision and smoothness of the execution of the intended action. Their function is the choice of an appropriate motor pattern and to globally organize the movements by reacting to affordances. The content of those intentions is not consciously accessible.

This threefold description of intentions is in line with our three-fold analysis of knowledge-formats: Obviously, D-intentions rely on the propositional, M-intentions on the nonconceptual sensorimotor format. Moreover, the intermediate P-intentions show the explanatory force of our third, i.e., the image-like knowledge format. It can't be assimilated to the abstract, propositional format since it is more fine-grained and relates to the particularities of our acting situations. However, it can't be reduced to the nonconceptual sensorimotor knowledge format either since it is consciously accessible and operating at a higher degree of abstraction.

In the same way as the reference to P-intentions is necessary to appropriately describe how we implement our rational intentions into a particular acting situation, the image-like knowledge format is necessary to bridge the gap between theoretical knowledge about our action, i.e., the explicit knowledge of the rules and criteria that guide of actions, to the practical knowledge, i.e., the successful performance of our intended actions.

5.9 Conclusion

We have argued that Ryle's approach to knowing-how and knowing-that crosses two different projects: the "semantic analysis" project, on the one hand, the "knowledge representation" projects. On the basis of this distinction we have characterized two kinds of intellectualism and shown that both show some severe problems: Whereas the first kind of intellectualism illegitimately neglects the pragmatics of our language use, the second one is not able to bridge the "Knowledge-Action-Gap". We have proposed a new framework by distinguishing two forms of knowledge (theoretical and practical) and three kinds of knowledge formats (propositional, nonconceptual sensorimotor, image-like).

We think that the discussion about knowing-how and knowing-that Ryle initiated should not be reduced to the conflict between intellectualism and anti-intellectualism since this discussion often relies on misunderstandings. Instead we should focus on some important questions Ryle raised, for example, how can we explain our ability to ride a bicycle? And how is our practical knowledge related to the things we know theoretically concerning riding a bike? We suggested a new conceptual framework that offers a starting point for convincing answers to these questions that touch on topics from various different disciplines as epistemology, philosophy of mind and action as well as the cognitive and neurosciences.

References

Adams, M.P. 2009. Empirical evidence and the knowledge-that/knowledge-how distinction. *Synthese* 170(1):97–114.

Anderson, J.R. 1980. *Cognitive Psychology and its Implications*. Freeman.

Bengson, J., M. Moffett, and J. Wright. 2009. The folk on "knowing how". *Philosophical Studies* 142:387–401.

Brinck, I. 1999. Nonconceptual content and the distinction between implicit and explicit knowledge. Commentary to Dienes & Perner. *Behavioral and Brain Sciences* 22(5):760–761.

Craig, E. 1990. *Knowledge and the State of Nature. An Essay in Conceptual Synthesis*. Oxford University Press.

Dienes, Z. and J. Perner. 1999. A theory of implicit and explicit knowledge. *Behavioral and Brain Sciences* 22:735–808.

Evans, G. 1982. *The Varieties of Reference*. Clarendon Press.

Eysenck, M.W., A. Ellis, E. Hunt, and P.N. Johnson-Laird, eds. 1994. *The Blackwell Dictionary of Cognitive Psychology*. Blackwell.

Fodor, J.A. 1968. The appeal to tacit knowledge in psychological explanation. *Journal of Philosophy* 65(20):627–640.

Fodor, J.A. 1978. Propositional attitudes. *The Monist* 61:501–523.

Fodor, J.A. 1998. *Concepts: Where Cognitive Science Went Wrong*. Oxford University Press.

Gibson, J.J. 1979. *The Ecological Approach to Visual Perception*. Houghton Mifflin.

Gunther, Y.H., ed. 2003. *Essays on Nonperceptual Content*. MIT Press.

Hanna, P. 2006. Swimming and speaking Spanish. *Philosophia* 34:267–285.

Hawley, K. 2003. Success and knowledge-how. *American Philosophical Quarterly* 40(1):19–31.

Hintikka, J. 1975. Different constuctions in terms of the basic epistemological verbs. A survey of some problems and proposals. In J. Hintikka, ed., *The Intentions of Intentionality and other new models for modalities*, pages 1–25. Reidel.

Hornsby, J. 2007. Knowledge and abilities in action. In C. Kanzian et al., ed., *Cultures. Conflict – analysis – dialogue. Proceedings of the 29th International Ludwig Wittgenstein-Symposium*, pages 165–180. Ontos.

Jeannerod, M. 1997. *The Cognitive Neuroscience of Action*. Blackwell.

Jung, E.-M. and A. Newen. 2010. Knowledge and abilities: The need for a new understanding of knowing-how. *Phenomenology and Cognitive Sciences* 9(1):113–131.

Markie, P. 2006. Knowing how is not knowing that. *Southwest Philosophy Review* 22(1):17–24.

Mechsner, F., D. Kerzel, G. Knoblich, and W. Prinz. 2001. Perceptual basis of bimanual coordination. *Nature* 414:69–73.

Mele, A.R. 1992. *Springs of Action: Understanding Intentional Behavior*. Oxford University Press.

Milner, A.D. and M.A. Goodale. 1993. Visual pathways to perception and action. In T. Hicks, S. Molotchnikoff, and T. Ono, eds., *Progress in Brain Research*, vol. 95, pages 317–337. Elsevier.

Müller, M. and R. Wehner. 1988. Path integration in desert ants, *Cataglyphis fortis. Proceedings of the National Academy of Sciences of the United States of America* 85(14):5287–5290.

Newen, A. 1997. The logic of indexical thoughts and the metaphysics of the "self". In W. Künne, A. Newen, and M. Anduschus, eds., *Reference, Indexicality and Propositional Attitudes*, pages 105–131. CSLI.

Newen, A. and A. Bartels. 2007. Animal minds and the possession of concepts. *Philosophical Psychology* 20(3):283–308.

Noë, A. 2005. Against intellectualism. *Analysis* 65:278–290.

Nozick, R. 1981. *Philosophical Explanations*. Harvard University Press.

Pacherie, E. 2008. The phenomenology of action: a conceptual framework,. *Cognition* 107(1):179–217.

Peacocke, C. 1992. *A Study of Concepts*. MIT Press.

Perry, J. 1979. The problem of the essential indexical. *Noûs* 13:3–21.

Poston, T. 2009. Know how to be gettiered? *Philosophy and Phenomenological Research* 79(3):743–747.

Rumfitt, I. 2003. Savoir faire. *Journal of Philosophy* 100:158–166.

Ryle, G. 1945. Knowing how and knowing that. *Proceedings of the Aristotelian Society* pages 1–16.

Ryle, G. 1949. *The Concept of Mind*. Rowman & Littlefield.

Sacks, O. 2007. *Musicophilia. Tales of Music and the Brain*. Random House.

Schack, T. and F. Mechsner. 2006. Representation of motor skills in human long-term memory. *Neuroscience Letters* 391:77–81.

Searle, J. 1983. *Intentionality: An Essay in the Philosophy of Mind*. Cambridge University Press.

Snowdon, P. 2004. Knowing how and knowing that: A distinction reconsidered. *Proceedings of the Aristotelian Society* 104(1):1–29.

Stanley, J. forthcoming. Knowing (how). *Noûs* no. doi: 10.1111/j.1468-0068.2010.00758.x:32 pages.

Stanley, J. and T. Williamson. 2001. Knowing how. *Journal of Philosophy* 98(8):411–444.

Stout, R. 2010. What you know when you know an answer to a question. *Noûs* 44(2):392–402.

White, A. 1982. *The Nature of Knowledge*. Rowman & Littlefield.

Zatorre, R.J. and A.R. Halpern. 2005. Mental concerts: Musical imagery and auditory cortex. *Neuron* 47:9–12.

Zatorre, R.J., A.R. Halpern, D.W. Perry, E. Meyer, and A.C. Evans. 1996. Hearing in the mind's ear: A PET investigation of musical imagery and perception. *Journal of Cognitive Neuroscience* 8:29–46.

Part II

Representation

6

Representation in Analog Computation

Gerard O'Brien & Jon Opie

6.1 Introduction

Not so long ago there was something of a consensus regarding the conceptual foundations of cognitive science. Participants in this multidisciplinary enterprise were united in the conviction that natural intelligence is to be explained in *computational* terms. Furthermore, since "there is no computation without representation" (Fodor 1975, 34), it seemed obvious that cognitive explanation requires *mental representation*. Computation and representation were the twin foundation stones on which the whole business was based (see, e.g., Thagard 2008).

These days things are very different. Representation is under attack from several quarters. There have always been sceptics about the prospects of naturalizing the mysterious "aboutness" of mental states, but attention has recently turned to concerns about the explanatory role of mental representation in cognitive science. Two lines of argument stand out. The first stems from the worry that semantic properties are, by nature, incapable of shaping cognitive processes. It was precisely this worry that prompted Stephen Stich (1983) to advocate replacing the computational theory of mind with the *syntactic* theory of mind. The second derives from the perceived failure of the computational theory of mind to deliver on its promise of explaining intelligence, and correlatively, the failure of traditional approaches in AI to construct deeply intelligent systems. Some theorists regard this problem as so

Knowledge and Representation.
Albert Newen, Andreas Bartels
& Eva-Maria Jung (eds.).
Copyright © 2011, CSLI Publications.

severe that cognitive science should abandon its flirtation with *representation*: "Representation is the wrong unit of abstraction in building the bulkiest parts of intelligent systems" (Brooks 1991, 140).

These arguments have begun to marginalise representation in cognitive science. There is talk of a Kuhnian-style paradigm shift in which the computational theory of mind will give way to *dynamical systems theory*, or some other approach that emphasises the *embodied* and *embedded* nature of cognition.[1] What unites these positions is scepticism about explaining intelligence in computational terms. Instead, cognition is conceived as a coupling between organism and environment, such that the world acts as its own representation (e.g., Brooks 1991, O'Regan and Noë 2001). This is an extraordinary situation, given the pivotal role of the concepts of representation and computation in the development of cognitive science.

We think this anti-representationalist movement marks a wrong turn in cognitive science. Without representation, cognitive science is bereft of its principal tool for explaining natural intelligence. It is thus incumbent on admirers of cognitive science to rescue representation from its threatened extinction. This chapter is written with that aim in mind.

Our diagnosis is that anti-representationalism has its roots in an overly restrictive take on mental representation that arose in the 1960s and 1970s. It was during this period that digital computers superseded analog computers, and in the process profoundly influenced our thinking about the mind. We will examine how digital computation has shaped our understanding of mental representation, and consider what cognitive science might have looked like had it arisen in the 1930s and 1940s, during the heyday of analog computation. Specifically, we will flesh out an account of representation based on careful analysis of the *Differential Analyzer*: the world's first general-purpose computer, and an analog device to boot. Our account undermines anti-representationalism, which turns out to be an attack on digital forms of representation, rather than representation *tout court*.

6.2   Revisiting the Foundations of Cognitive Science

The birth of cognitive science (and its technology-focused fellow traveller, the field of artificial intelligence) is often identified with the Dartmouth conference of 1956.[2] Whether or not such a specific dating is possible, what was ultimately responsible for establishing the field was

---

[1]See, e.g., Beer (1995), Brooks (1991), Clark (1997a,b), Keijzer (2002), Port and van Gelder (1995), van Gelder (1995), Wallace et al. (2007), Wheeler (2005).

[2]See, e.g., Copeland (1993), 8.

a series of intellectual and technical achievements during the 1950s and 1960s. Noam Chomsky's (1959) lacerating critique of B. F. Skinner's *Verbal Behavior* is among the former, because it sounded the death knell for the behaviourism that had dominated psychology in the first half of the twentieth century. And chief among the latter was the rapid development of the electronic digital computer. A number of important innovations took place at this time, including the development of the von Neumann, stored-program architecture. But the efflorescence of digital computers was largely the result of a technical breakthrough— the introduction of the transistor as the basic computing element. As a result, digital computers were immediately smaller, faster, cheaper to produce, and more reliable.

So when cognitive scientists first proposed that cognition is computation, it's no surprise they turned to the theory of digital computers to flesh out this conjecture. To solve a problem by digital means one first develops a *formal description* of the problem domain, and then *physically implements* that description. A formal description comprises a set of symbols that represent the elements of the target domain, together with syntactic rules that describe the behaviour of those elements. A physical implementation of a formal description consists of a device whose internal states realize the symbols in the description, and whose state-transitions satisfy the syntactic rules.[3]

When cognitive science looked to computer science for a model of cognition, it was this familiar picture of rule-governed symbol manipulation that emerged. And despite various developments in cognitive science since that time, including the appearance of connectionism in the 1980s, this conception of cognition has stuck.

However, the history of computer science has *two* strands: digital and analog. Digital computing has its origin in the methods of arithmetic. The first digital computers were devices such as the abacus, which appeared in Babylonia around 300 BC. Analog computation originated with *non-symbolic* graphical and geometric methods. The earliest known analog computer—the Antikythera mechanism, used to calculate astronomical positions—was built in about 100 BC (Bromley 1990). During the 1930s and 1940s, computer science was dominated by mechanical analog computers. And contrary to the popular view that analog computers are all "special-purpose" devices, the first general-purpose, automatic computer was actually an analog machine:

---

[3] Haugeland (1985) is the classic philosophical account of formal descriptions and their physical realization.

the Differential Analyzer developed by Vannevar Bush at MIT in the 1930s.

The rapid advance of electronic technology during the Second World War enabled digital computers to perform numerical calculations at speeds sufficient to rival analog devices. But it wasn't until the 1960s, with the dramatic reduction in costs that accompanied the development of transistorised circuits, that digital computers largely supplanted analog devices. Indeed, prior to this time, analog computers were often preferred, particularly in applications where accurate real-time calculations were required (Small 1993).

Given that the emergence of digital computation is best explained as a result of a technical innovation, rather than a conceptual revolution, it is worth considering what cognitive science might have looked like had it been founded on an analog conception of cognition. In particular, what account of representation might have emerged from the analog computational framework? In the next section we will start to explore this question by revisiting the distinction between analog and digital computation.

6.3 Distinguishing between Digital and Analog Computation

The relationship between digital and analog computation is subject to some confusion. It's often claimed that the essential difference between the two is that digital computers use *discrete* variables to represent their targets (e.g., high and low voltage states), whereas analog computers use *continuous* variables. This way of dividing things up appears to be based on the view that a physical system performs a computation just in case its operation can be interpreted as implementing some function. Churchland et al. (1993) express the idea as follows:

> [W]e can consider a physical system as a computational system just in case there is an appropriate (revealing) mapping between some algorithm and associated physical variables. More exactly, a physical system computes a function $f(x)$ when there is (1) a mapping between the system's physical inputs and x, (2) a mapping between the system's physical outputs and y, such that (3) $f(x) = y$. (Churchland et al. 1993, 48)

This view of computation suggests the following way of distinguishing between digital and analog computers: a physical system is a digital computer if its state variables map onto a discrete function, an analog computer if its state variables map onto a continuous function. Despite the tidiness of this scheme, and a certain degree of acceptance within the computer science community, we believe this way of proceeding is deeply mistaken. It fails on two grounds.

First, there is good reason to reject the idea that computation is merely a matter of implementing a function. Since all law-governed physical systems can be interpreted as implementing some function or other, this view leads to the conclusion that *all* physical systems are computational. But the concept of computation was originally introduced into cognitive science as a way of distinguishing two classes of causal processes: those characteristic of systems (such as ovens, cups of tea, and cyclones) that show no signs of intelligence, and those exhibited by intelligent systems alone. Computational processes are supposed to be *special* in some way—in a way, moreover, that provides us with some explanatory purchase on the problem of intelligent behaviour. Implementing a function is a ubiquitous feature of nature, so characterizing computation in this way undermines the motivation for introducing the concept in the first place.[4]

Secondly, recourse to the divide between discrete and continuous variables is at odds with the way computer scientists themselves have generally drawn the analog/digital distinction. Consider, for example, the familiar tactic of representing a physical variable as a curve on the plane. If we plot the velocity of a moving object against time, it is possible to compute the distance it travels by measuring the area under the curve, or its acceleration at some instant by constructing a tangent to the curve (Figure 1 on the next page).

These computations employ an *analog* representing vehicle, a 2-d curve plotted against a pair of linear axes. What makes this representation analog is the existence of a relation-preserving mapping between the curve and its target. Velocity is represented as the projection of the curve onto the y-axis, such that relations among velocities correspond to relations among those points. If the velocity at some time t_3 is greater than the velocity at t_1, then its representative point v_3 will be further along the vertical axis than v_1; if the velocity at t_2 is mid-way between the first two velocities, then v_2 will lie between v_1 and v_3, and so on (Figure 1 on the following page). In other words, there is a simple *physical analogy* between the curve and the variable it represents. Such analogies are responsible for the effectiveness of both special-purpose analog devices, such as scale models, and general purpose analog computers such as the Differential Analyzer (as we will demonstrate).

---

[4]For further discussion see O'Brien and Opie (2006). We there suggest an alternative characterization of computation that avoids this criticism.

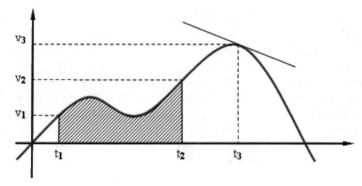

FIGURE 1 A graph of velocity versus time. The distance travelled between t_1 and t_2 can be computed by measuring the area of the shaded region. The acceleration at t_3 can be computed by measuring the slope of the tangent to the curve at that point.

Classic texts in engineering and computer science such as Jackson (1960), Truitt and Rogers (1960), and Soroka (1954) make precisely this point.

> Devices that rely ... on the analogous relationships that subsist between the physical quantities associated with a computer and the quantities associated with a problem under study are called *analog* computers. (Jackson 1960, 1)

> All [analog computers] have one characteristic in common—that the components of each computer ... are assembled to permit the computer to perform as a model, or in a manner analogous to some other physical system. (Truitt and Rogers 1960, 3)

> The term *analog* means similarity of properties or relations without identity. When analogous systems are found to exist, measurements or other observations made on one of these systems may be used to predict the behaviour of the others. (Soroka 1954, v)

What these authors are suggesting is that an analog computer is a device designed to exploit an analogy between the physical properties of a system of representing vehicles and some target system. Digital computers don't work that way, instead deploying symbolic vehicles whose physical properties stand in an arbitrary relationship to the objects they represent.[5] The distinction between continuous and discrete vari-

---

[5]This implies that symbols don't carry their meaning intrinsically, but acquire meaning by virtue of how they are manipulated. For example, numerals represent numbers not because of their physical form, but because we operate on them according to syntactic rules that support a numerical interpretation. See Section 6.5 for further details.

ables is not fundamental to the relationship between analog and digital computation, because analog representation need not involve continuous variables. Modern analog clocks, for example, represent time via the angular position of hands on a dial. But such clocks typically represent time to a resolution of no better than a second, because their hands move in *discrete* steps around the dial.[6]

6.4   The Differential Analyzer

Most early analog computers were special-purpose devices. They were designed to perform computations related to a particular problem or system. For example, during the 1870s Lord Kelvin invented an analog device that determined the components of tidal variation by performing a Fourier analysis of tide height records. Kelvin's *Harmonic Analyzer* used a system of disk-and-ball integrators developed by his brother James Thomson (Bromley 1990, 172–4). In the 1910s and 1920s, Hannibal Ford produced a number of very accurate analog computers for determining the range of moving targets. These were used extensively in ship-to-ship naval gunnery and later for anti-aircraft fire control (Clymer 1993). But these sophisticated mechanical computers were designed with a narrow range of applications in mind. Scientists and engineers, who sought to develop mathematical models unhindered by the limits of analytic techniques, were sorely in need of general-purpose computers.

In 1876, Kelvin discovered that by creating a feedback connection between two integrators he could solve linear second-order differential equations. He also saw how to generalize the feedback principle to differential equations of any order, but technical difficulties prevented him from constructing a working model (Bromley 1990, 174–7). Fifty years later, Vannevar Bush and his students independently developed an electromechanical device capable of solving second-order equations. Again, the original impetus had been to solve equations connected with specific physical systems,[7] but the result was a general-purpose device. Like Kelvin, Bush was aware of the need to generalize to higher-order systems of equations. The key to Bush's success was the introduction of mechanical torque amplifiers (a suggestion of his student Harold Hazen) and highly accurate disk-and-wheel integrators. Torque amplifiers permit a series of integrators to drive one another despite their inherently limited output—the very problem that had hindered Kelvin's work (Owens 1986, 66–70). With these innovations in place, Bush and

---

[6]See Lewis (1971) for further examples of discrete analog representation.

[7]Among other things, Bush and his students investigated long-distance transmission lines and vacuum-tube circuits. See Owens (1986), 66–70, for further details.

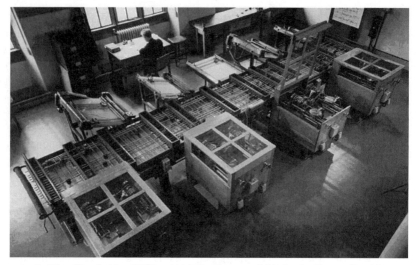

FIGURE 2 The Cambridge Differential Analyzer, which is similar to Bush's design. The disk-and-wheel integrators are on the right; the input and output tables on the left.

his colleagues were able to build the first *Differential Analyzer*, a mechanical analog computer capable of quickly and accurately solving differential equations of any desired order.

Bush's computer consisted of a long table criss-crossed by a series of rotating shafts (Figure 2). On one side of the table were six disk-and-wheel integrators interlinked by torque amplifiers. On the opposite side were a set of boards, some used to graph output variables, others to generate input via an operator who traced a graph of the input function, thereby governing the rotation of a shaft. Each shaft was associated with a variable, and by using geared connections between them it was possible to add, subtract, multiply, divide and integrate variables.

The heart of a Differential Analyzer is the disk-and-wheel integrator. This device takes any variable as input and produces its integral as output. It consists of a metal disk, and a small wheel oriented at right angles to the disk such that rotation of the disk causes the wheel to rotate. The wheel is also free to move along the radius of the disk, its position determined by the lateral movement of a connecting shaft (Figure 3 on the facing page). Suppose the disk turns through the angle Δx. If the radius of the wheel is r and its distance from the centre of the disk is f, then:

$$f\Delta x = r\Delta y$$

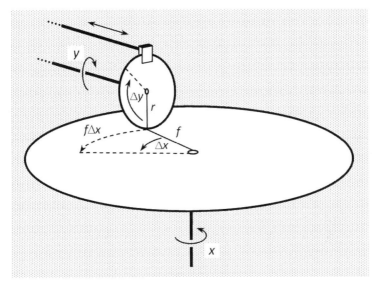

FIGURE 3 A disk-and-wheel integrator. The small wheel rotates in response to rotation of the disk, and is free to move along the radius of the disk as a result of linear movements of the upper shaft. The figure is modified by J. Opie on the basis of Bromley (1990).

This expresses the fact that the length of the path traced out on the disk by the rotating wheel must equal the arc on the wheel itself. In the Differential Analyzer the rotation of the disk indirectly governs the lateral movement of the wheel (see below for details), so f is actually a function of x. Rearranging and taking the limit for small Δx we get:

$$f = r\frac{dy}{dx}$$

That is, f is proportional to the derivative of y with respect to x. For a unit wheel, this implies:

$$y(t) - y(0) = \int_0^t f(x)\,dx$$

In other words, the angular displacement Δy of the wheel is the integral of the function that describes the linear motion of the upper shaft. Depending on one's interests one might therefore describe the disk-and-wheel system as a *model* of the integration process, or a *means of calculating* the integral of a function.

To illustrate how a Differential Analyzer works, consider the problem of modelling an object in free fall near the surface of the earth. Such an object is subject to two forces: the force of gravity, and an opposing force caused by air resistance which is proportional to the object's velocity. The acceleration of the object is given by:

(1) $$\frac{d^2y}{dt^2} = g - k\frac{dy}{dt}$$

Here g is the acceleration due to gravity and k is a drag coefficient. To solve Equation (1), the Differential Analyzer is set up as shown in Figure 4 on the facing page. Each shaft represents a variable or constant in the equation. The first lengthwise shaft is driven at a constant rate, so its angular position is a suitable representation of time. It acts like a metronome, tapping out a beat that is followed by the rest of the system. The next three shafts represent acceleration d^2y/dt^2, velocity dy/dt, and position y, respectively. Both integrators are driven by the time shaft. The acceleration shaft (shaft 2) determines the linear motion of the wheel on the first integrator, so its output is:

(2) $$\frac{dy}{dt} = \int \frac{d^2y}{dt^2}\, dt$$

The velocity shaft (shaft 3) determines the linear motion of the wheel on the second integrator. Its output is position, because:

(3) $$y = \int \frac{dy}{dt}\, dt$$

The last two shafts (5 and 6) represent the product of velocity and the drag coefficient, and the acceleration due to gravity, respectively. They are added by a crucial set of connections which provide input to the acceleration shaft, as per Equation (1). To solve Equation (1) one initializes the shafts and turns on the driving motor. A graph of position versus time will immediately begin to appear on the plotting table, and it is this graph that constitutes a solution to the equation.

It is noteworthy that the operation of this system is *completely parallel*, in the sense that every variable is generated *simultaneously*. The instant the time shaft begins to rotate, this motion is communicated to the integrators, the first of which calculates velocity, the second, position, taking velocity as its input. Because the components of the system are rigidly connected, there is virtually no delay between these events and the moment when the sum of the final two shafts starts to provide feedback to the acceleration shaft. Although the free-fall equation can be solved using formal methods, the Differential Analyzer produces a solution very rapidly, and can with equal facility solve equations for which no exact formal solution exists.

So how and in what sense does this device compute a solution to the free-fall equation? Certainly not in the manner of a digital computer,

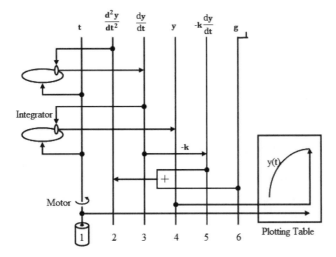

FIGURE 4 A Differential Analyzer set up to solve the free-fall equation.
Each shaft represents a variable or a constant in the equation. The analyzer
requires two integrators because it is designed to solve a second-order
differential equation. The first lengthwise shaft is driven by a motor at a
constant speed and represents the independent variable t. The figure is
modified by J. Opie on the basis of Bromley (1990).

which instantiates a set of formal rules designed to govern the transformation of numerical symbols. Here there are no formal rules, and no
symbols. Instead, the Differential Analyzer is "an elegant, dynamical,
mechanical model of the differential equation" (Owens 1986, 75, emphasis added). Describing the analyzer in this way is appropriate when
our target is a mathematical problem. But it can equally be described
as a model of an object in free fall. Under either description, the analyzer computes a solution by producing an output that represents the
variable of interest to us.[8] And it does so because its own operations
are described by Equation (1) on the facing page. The classic texts in
computer science are again clear on this point:

> [T]he analog-computer family consists of all those devices in which
> measurable physical quantities are made to obey mathematical re-
> lationships comparable with those existing in a particular problem.
> (Smith and Wood 1959, 1)

---

[8]Note that the analyzer of Figure 4 can easily be modified to output a graph of
velocity or acceleration.

> Analog models are devices that behave in a fashion analogous to others simply because they obey the same or similar fundamental laws of nature. (Truitt and Rogers 1960, 7)

The analyzer models an equation by mechanically acting it out. This does not apply to a digital computer, whose governing equations are, in most cases, those that apply to the components of a digital electronic device. A digital computer models a target system by "running the maths", that is, by numerically calculating the values of a function that describes the system. It does not itself obey those equations.

6.5 Representation in Analog Computation

The Differential Analyzer was the first general purpose analog computer. It was followed in the 1950s and 1960s by a series of increasingly sophisticated electronic computers, which employed electronic counterparts of the analyzer's adders, multipliers, integrators, and so on (Small 1993). Such computers were initially less accurate than their mechanical brethren, but cheaper to build and easier to program (Bromley 1990). Like the Differential Analyzer, they were general purpose analog devices that could be used to model a wide variety of systems by combining components as required (Truitt and Rogers 1960).

Analog computers of all stripes operate in conformity with the equations they are designed to solve. We claimed in Section 6.3 that such systems exploit a physical analogy between a system of representing vehicles and the objects they represent. In this section we will consider what this implies about analog representation, using the Differential Analyzer as our touchstone.

Scientists who worked with Differential Analyzers took it for granted that they could be used to represent physical or mathematical objects. Representations are *content-bearers*: things that carry meaning. Although a completely general account of representation still eludes us, there is some consensus that such an account must address two main questions:

- *The Role Question.* What systemic role must something fill to *be* a representation, i.e., what makes some state or object a content-bearer in the first place?
- *The Content Question.* What determines the content of a representation?

It is commonplace these days for theorists to insist that any answer to the role question must emphasize the place of "interpretation". Bits of the world only become representations when there is some *user* for whom they operate as content bearers.[9] Digital and analog computers are alike in this regard: both digital and analog representation is always representation *for* or *to* some further system or process. But despite this common ground, digital and analog computers differ crucially with respect to the content question.

Symbols stand in an *arbitrary* physical relationship to the things they represent. Consequently, the content of the representations in a digital computer cannot be determined by their intrinsic properties. The standard story is that this content emerges as a result of the computational processes in which such representations are implicated.[10] In a modern electronic calculator, for example, the internal circuitry is so arranged that transitions among select groups of voltage states conform to the rules that regulate arithmetic. And it is this internal causal organization that licenses the interpretation of the voltage states as representing specific numbers.

Analog computers, on the other hand, are designed to exploit an analogy between the physical properties of a system of representing vehicles and some target system. This entails that analog representations, by contrast with symbols, stand in a *non-arbitrary* physical relationship to the things they represent. The content of analog representations is determined by certain of their intrinsic properties—those that ground the physical analogy between the computer and the system it represents.

Consider the Differential Analyzer we described in Section 6.4. The physical analogy between this analyzer and an object in free fall is captured formally by Equation (1) on page 118, but to fully appreciate this relationship one needs to understand the dynamics of the two systems. When first released, an object falling near the surface of the earth has an acceleration $g = 9.8\,\mathrm{ms}^{-2}$. Such an object quickly picks up speed, but the faster it falls, the more drag it experiences. Eventually the object's acceleration will reduce to zero, at which point it reaches its terminal velocity. Equation (1) describes the relationship between linear acceleration and velocity that results from these forces. But equally, Equation (1) describes the behaviour of our Differential Analyzer. In this case, the variable y corresponds to the angular position of shaft 4.

---

[9]Peirce (1955) argued long ago that representation is a triadic relation between a representing vehicle, a represented object, and an "interpretant". Others who have emphasised the triadic nature of representation are Millikan (1984), whose "representation-consumers" correspond to Peirce's "interpretants", Bechtel (1998, 2009), and O'Brien and Opie (2004).

[10]The standard story is disputed by some theorists, most famously by Jerry Fodor (see, e.g., Fodor 1987).

This shaft rotates in a manner that is analogous to the behaviour of an object in free fall. It begins at rest, but then begins to rotate with an angular acceleration equal to the constant g (set by the position of shaft 6), and a steadily increasing angular velocity. Its acceleration gradually reduces as a result of feedback from shaft 5, which mimics the effect of drag, and hence its angular velocity will reach a "terminal" value. The mechanical principles that give rise to this behaviour are those of a device incorporating two integrators (as described in Section 6.4) and the set of gearings and connections portrayed in Figure 4 on page 119.

So our Differential Analyzer can be used to model an object in free fall precisely because the rotational dynamics of its "position" shaft (shaft 4) is physically analogous to the linear dynamics of an object in free fall. The angular position of shaft 4 and the displacement of a falling object are in fact *isomorphic*. Formally, this means that there is a relation-preserving mapping from angular position onto displacement. Informally, it means that the graphs of these two variables have the same shape, and overlap if placed one on top of the other. Thus, the graph produced by our Differential Analyzer is at once a record of the behaviour of shaft four, and a representation of the motion of an object falling near the surface of the earth.

Physical analogy is a *resemblance relation*. Two systems resemble each other if they share first-order properties, such as mass or conductivity, or second-order properties, such as layout or organization. A nice example of second-order resemblance is the relationship between the width of a tree's growth rings and seasonal rainfall. Plentiful seasons produce wide rings, whereas drought years produce comparatively narrow rings. For this reason, if we map the set of growth rings (indexed by year) into the set of seasons, variations in rainfall are reflected in the relative width of the rings.[11] When a second-order resemblance is grounded in properties or relations that are *intrinsic* to some material system, as in this case, it is a physical analogy. Other physical analogies include the relationships between: (i) a land map and the terrain it portrays, (ii) the mercury levels in a thermometer and ambient temperature, and (iii) the movements of the dial on a kitchen scale and the masses it registers. In each of these cases we harness a second-order physical analogy for representational purposes. A thermometer can be used to represent temperature because one of its intrinsic properties

---

[11]This mapping is unlikely to be an isomorphism, because the width of tree rings only approximately corresponds to variations in the weather. But even when the mapping between the parts and relations of two systems is patchy and inexact, we may still legitimately speak of them resembling each other.

(the height of the mercury) bears a non-arbitrary relationship to that variable.

What the foregoing makes clear is that the representational content of a Differential Analyzer, and our free-fall analyzer in particular, depends on a physical analogy between the analyzer and its target. In the next and final section we consider what implications this might have for cognitive science.

6.6 Representation Redux

The current disquiet about mental representation depends on two main lines of argument. The first begins with the premise that the specifically semantic properties of representing vehicles are by nature incapable of shaping cognition. The second, with the claim that cognitive science has by and large failed to explain the kind of fluid, context-sensitive intelligence exhibited by human beings and many other organisms. Both conclude that mental representation fails to earn its explanatory keep in cognitive science, and is best abandoned.

However, as we observed in Section 6.2, cognitive science grew up in an era when digital computers were in the ascendant. The heyday of analog computation was already over, and it was the theory of digital computation that shaped the thinking of the first cognitive scientists. Consequently, the dominant picture of mental representation ever since has been the one suggested by digital computation: mental representations are *symbols*. In our view, it is this picture of mental representation that has led to the marginalisation of representation in contemporary cognitive science.

A symbol, like any representation, has both intrinsic properties and semantic properties. The representational content of a symbol depends on the causal organization of the digital computer in which it is embedded. Machine states become symbols, as opposed to meaningless bits of syntax, if their behaviour is regulated by physically implemented transition rules that conform to an intended interpretation. But the intrinsic properties of a symbol have no direct bearing on its meaning. Consequently, the causal impact of a symbol on computational processes is not determined by its representational content.[12] This feature of digital computation has led to considerable controversy about the significance of representation for cognition, and to the view that representational content is at best merely "explanatorily relevant" to cognition.[13] Little

---

[12] The relationship between content and causation is in fact the reverse. It is the causal role of a symbol that determines its content.

[13] See, for example, Baker (1993), Fodor (1989), Jackson and Pettit (1990), and LePore and Loewer (1989).

wonder then, that Stich (1983) and others countenance dispensing with the computational perspective altogether.

As for deep intelligence, here the so-called "knowledge problem" looms large—the problem of equipping a cognitive system with the informational resources to choose appropriate courses of action in real time, in response to open-ended internal goals (Dennett 1984). This problem has stymied the best attempts of classical AI to produce fluid, human-like intelligence. One plausible analysis of this failure is that it represents a limitation inherent in classical AI's commitment to symbolic representation. We noted in Section 6.2 that to solve a problem by digital means one must physically implement a formal description of the problem domain. Because the symbols composing the formal description bear arbitrary relations to the elements of the modelled domain, the former can capture the latter only when their behaviour is disciplined by carefully crafted syntactic rules. As a consequence, representation in a digital computer inevitably has a "micro-managed" character, in the sense that each and every semantic relation among its symbols must be regulated by proprietary syntactic machinery. Moreover, whenever descriptive components are added to the formalism or existing components are updated (as is necessary in modelling the real world), a myriad of further rules must be installed to ensure continued semantic coherence. As the formalism grows richer in content, the number of rules, and with it the number of individual processing steps, increases dramatically. In a digital system operating in real-time, the representational demands quickly outstrip the processing capacities of even the fastest hardware.

How would cognitive science look if our conception of mental representation had been shaped by experience with analog computers? The answer, we contend, is that the field's recent flirtation with anti-representationalism would not have occurred. This is because the two principal arguments that have led to the marginalisation of representation in contemporary cognitive science gain no traction when viewed from the perspective of analog computation.

First, we've seen that analog computation, unlike its digital counterpart, is directly shaped by the content-determining properties of its vehicles. Since the representational content of a symbol is determined by factors extrinsic to that vehicle, its content can have no bearing on what it does. The representing vehicles in an analog computer, by contrast, acquire content by virtue of their intrinsic physical properties and the resemblance relations these support. Hence, the computational processes that occur in an analog computer are driven by the very properties that determine the content of its vehicles. In this sense, an analog computer is not a mere semblance of a semantic engine—it's the real thing. Any organism whose inner processes are analog in nature is causally indebted to the semantic properties of its inner states.

Second, the constraint that makes the knowledge problem so acute for digital computers—viz., that syntactic rules are required to discipline the causal commerce between symbols—doesn't apply to analog computers. An analog computer is powered by a physical analogy between its representing vehicles and its task domain. As a consequence, representation in an analog computer has an "autonomous" character, in the sense that the semantic relations among its representing vehicles are inherently aligned with their physical relations. So when the content of an analog computer is augmented, via the enrichment of the physical analogy between its representational medium and its target domain, the semantic relations among its constituent vehicles take care of themselves. *Prima facie*, analog computers have the potential to capture the real-world, real-time character of deep intelligence.

From this perspective, contemporary anti-representationalism is best understood as a reaction to the *symbolic* form of representation implicated in digital computation, rather than *representation per se*. Cognitive science grew up at a time when digital computers, largely on the back of technical innovations, had supplanted their analog brethren. Digital computers have dominated and conditioned theorising in the field ever since. But digital computers have limitations—limitations owing to the fact that they are not genuine semantic engines, but ingeniously crafted syntactic devices that behave *as if* they were semantic engines. Instead of responding to these limitations by ditching representation and entertaining alternatives to computation, as many in the field are doing, the analysis we have presented suggests it would be more fruitful for cognitive science to explore the alternative *form* of computation.

References

Baker, L.R. 1993. Metaphysics and mental causation. In J. Heil and A. Mele, eds., *Mental Causation*. Oxford University Press.

Bechtel, W. 1998. Representations and cognitive explanations: Assessing the dynamicist's challenge in cognitive science. *Cognitive Science* 22:295–318.

Bechtel, W. 2009. Constructing a philosophy of science of cognitive science. *Topics in Cognitive Science* 1:548–569.

Beer, R.D. 1995. A dynamical systems perspective on agent-environment interaction. *Artificial Intelligence* 72(1-2):173–215.

Bromley, A.G. 1990. Analog computing devices. In W. Aspray, ed., *Computing Before Computers*. Iowa Sate Press.

Brooks, A. 1991. Intelligence without representation. *Artificial Intelligence* 47:139–59.

Chomsky, N. 1959. Review of Skinner's "Verbal Behavior". *Language* 35:26–58.

Churchland, P., C. Koch, and T. Sejnowski. 1993. What is computational neuroscience? In E. Schwartz, ed., *Computational Neuroscience*. MIT Press.

Clark, A. 1997a. *Being There: Putting Brain, Body and World Together Again*. MIT Press.

Clark, A. 1997b. The dynamical challenge. *Cognitive Science* 21:461–81.

Clymer, A.B. 1993. The mechanical analog computers of Hannibal Ford and William Newell. *IEEE Annals of the History of Computing* 15(2):9–34.

Copeland, B.J. 1993. *Artificial Intelligence: A Philosophical Introduction*. Wiley-Blackwell.

Dennett, D.C. 1984. Cognitive wheels: The frame problem of AI. In C. Hookway, ed., *Minds, Machines and Evolution*. Cambridge University Press.

Fodor, J.A. 1975. *The Language of Thought*. Harvester Press.

Fodor, J.A. 1987. *Psychosemantics: The Problem of Meaning in the Philosophy of Mind*. MIT Press.

Fodor, J.A. 1989. Making mind matter more. *Philosophical Topics* 17:59–79.

Haugeland, J. 1985. *Artificial Intelligence: The Very Idea*. MIT Press.

Jackson, A.S. 1960. *Analog Computation*. McGraw-Hill.

Jackson, F. and P. Pettit. 1990. Program explanation: A general perspective. *Analysis* 50:107–117.

Keijzer, F. 2002. Representation in dynamical and embodied cognition. *Systems Research* 3:275–288.

LePore, E. and B. Loewer. 1989. More on making mind matter. *Philosophical Topics* 17:175–191.

Lewis, D. 1971. Analog and digital. *Noûs* 5:321–327.

Millikan, R.G. 1984. *Language, thought, and other biological categories*. MIT Press.

O'Brien, G. and J. Opie. 2004. Notes towards a structuralist theory of mental representation. In H. Clapin, P. Staines, and P. Slezak, eds., *Representation in Mind: New Approaches to Mental Representation*. Elsevier.

O'Brien, G. and J. Opie. 2006. How do connectionist networks compute? *Cognitive Processing* 7:30–41.

O'Regan, J.K. and A. Noë. 2001. A sensorimotor account of vision and visual consciousness. *Behavioral and Brain Sciences* 24:939–1031.

Owens, L. 1986. Vannevar Bush and the Differential Analyzer: The text and context of an early computer. *Technology and Culture* 27(1):63–95.

Peirce, C.S. 1955. Logic as semiotic: The theory of signs. In J. Buchler, ed., *Philosophical Writings of Peirce*. Dover Publications.

Port, R. and T. van Gelder. 1995. *Mind as Motion: Explorations in the Dynamics of Cognition*. MIT Press.

Small, J.S. 1993. General-purpose electronic analog computing: 1945–1965. *IEEE Annals of the History of Computing* 15(2):8–18.

Smith, G.W. and R.C. Wood. 1959. *Principles of Analog Computation*. McGraw-Hill.

Soroka, W. 1954. *Analog Methods in Computation and Simulation*. McGraw-Hill.

Stich, S. 1983. *From Folk Psychology to Cognitive Science: The Case Against Belief*. MIT Press.

Thagard, P. 2008. Cognitive science. In E. Zalta, ed., *The Stanford Encyclopedia of Philosophy*. http://plato.stanford.edu/archives/fall2008/entries/cognitive-science/.

Truitt, T.D. and A.E. Rogers. 1960. *Basics of Analog Computers*. John F. Rider.

van Gelder, T. 1995. What might cognition be, if not computation? *Journal of Philosophy* 92:345–381.

Wallace, B., A. Ross, J. Davies, and T. Anderson, eds. 2007. *Mind, the Body and the World. Psychology after Cognitivism*. Imprint Academic.

Wheeler, M. 2005. *Reconstructing the Cognitive World: The Next Step*. MIT Press.

7

Representing Time of Day in Circadian Clocks

WILLIAM BECHTEL

7.1 Introduction

Positing representations and operations on them as a way of explaining behavior was one of the major innovations of the cognitive revolution. Neuroscience and biology more generally also employ representations in explaining how organisms function and coordinate their behavior with the world around them. In discussions of the nature of representation, theorists commonly differentiate between the vehicles of representation and their content—what they denote. Many contentious debates in cognitive science, such as those pitting neural network models against symbol processing accounts, have focused on the types of *vehicles* proposed for mental representation and whether they have the appropriate structure to succeed in bearing their contents. Philosophers, in contrast, have focused their debates on *content* and the particular way in which vehicles might bear content—that is, the process of representing rather than the format of representations. I will offer a novel answer to the question of how it is that a representation has content by focusing on the architecture of representation. My proposal is that representations occur in a particular type of mechanism—one in which a control system regulates a plant—and that we can gain traction on representations in cognitive systems by considering how this works in physical systems more generally.

Knowledge and Representation.
Albert Newen, Andreas Bartels
& Eva-Maria Jung (eds.).
Copyright © 2011, CSLI Publications.

Questions of representation, especially with respect to the content of mental representations, have a long and rather inconclusive history in philosophy. The simplest construal of content will be sufficient for my purposes here, namely, that the content of a representation is what it refers to, typically something in the external world. More challenging is the question of how representations come to have content. Philosophical accounts have tended to approach the problem in one of two ways. The first approach, seeking to capture the idea that representations carry information about what produced them, focuses on the role of the referent in generating the occurrence of the representation (Dretske 1981). One challenge is that representations can misrepresent by being about something other than what caused their occurrence. This led Brentano (1874) to suggest that intentionality (the relation between a representation and its content) is not a proper relation; others, though, have proposed a variety of solutions that preserve treating representing as involving a relation to a content. The second approach focuses on the consumer of the representation—the entity or system that uses the representation to secure information about its referent. The challenge for this approach is specifying what the system is treating as the content. A major proponent, Millikan (1984), appeals to natural selection to settle this question: the representation has a particular content because the representation itself was selected for its success in representing that content. Such an appeal to natural selection to ground representations has been challenged by Fodor (1990), who proposed his own alternative, and active debate continues among advocates of these various ways of explaining how representations have content.

In this paper I will not enter into the details of this debate, but advance an alternative account that situates both the focus on information and that on the consumer in a context that is actually motivated, ironically, by theorists who present themselves as rejecting appeals to representations in understanding the mind. Advocating a dynamical approach to cognitive science, van Gelder (1995) argued that, just like a much simpler dynamical system—the steam engine governor designed by James Watt—mental systems perform their tasks without representations. I concur with van Gelder that the Watt governor is a more productive model for understanding cognitive systems than is the digital computer widely invoked by theorists advancing representational accounts of the mind. But I will further argue that, properly understood, the Watt governor employs representations. The Watt governor is a control system, and like any other control system must employ representations to perform its task. A control system is part of a larger system and is specialized to regulate the behavior of other parts of that system. Often the part performing the control function is called the *controller* and the parts it controls the *plant*. The controller has internal operations that, when the system is functioning correctly, carry information about parts of the plant or entities or processes external to the plant that affect it. This information, whether it misrepresents or accurately represents actual states or activities, is used by the controller to regulate the plant's behavior.[1]

My main objective is to illustrate the value of thinking of representations and their content from this perspective. Rather than starting with representations as they might figure in cognitive accounts of activities such as reasoning or memory, though, I will focus on representations as described in neuroscience (and biology more generally), where we can more readily gain traction in accounting for their content. Neuroscientists have long characterized the brain processes they study as representational, but have left implicit the reasons for bringing in talk of representations. In Section 7.2 I note highlights of research on the primate visual system and show that the assumed framework is that of Dretske, according to which a neural process represents the stimulus that caused it. Neuroscientists are well aware, though, that neural processes may misrepresent stimuli; for example, in cases of illusions they characterize the mind as representing what the organism takes to exist in the world (vs. what actually exists). The framework of control theory provides a way of understanding this practice, so in Section 7.3 I take up the challenge posed by the dynamicists by showing how control systems require representations, albeit ones understood dynamically. In the remaining sections, I illustrate the control theory approach to understanding representations by focusing on a specific example: the circadian clocks by which organisms represent both time of day and the length of daylight (the photoperiod). Circadian clocks are physiological oscillators with a period of approximately 24 hours localized within individual cells (although often involving coordinated interactions among those cells). Research has revealed not only the basic mechanisms operating as circadian clocks within cells, but also has begun to shed light on how they can be entrained by time and length of day and can be used by other systems within the organism to regulate

---

[1]An advantage of this approach over that of Millikan is that it obviates any need to appeal to the history of the system to evaluate what are representations. If a system has a controller within it, the operations that carry information in that controller are representations, regardless of whether such processes were the product of selection at some point in the past. That is, even if a controller evolved via drift or some other non-selectionist process, its internal states count as representations. Whether something is a representation is a question about the role it plays within a system (does it figure in control processes?), not about its history.

behavior that depends upon time and length of day. I will not in this paper be able to extend the account into more cognitive domains, but presume that if an account succeeds in explaining how neural processes such as those involved in controlling circadian behavior have content, it can be extended to the processes the brain employs when engaged in tasks that are more clearly cognitive such as problem solving and making evaluative judgments.[2]

7.2 The Widespread Use of Representations in Neuroscience

In the 19th century, researchers began trying to localize responsibility for control of motor and sensory processing in the brain. Gall (1812) was an early pioneer, but his contemporaries severely challenged both his criteria for localization (correlations between the size of brain regions and behavioral propensities) and his implementation (using skull protrusions as a proxy for the size of a brain region, and positing correlations impressionistically rather than quantitatively). This led researchers in subsequent decades to be skittish about advancing similar claims. Broca's (1861) linkage of acquired speech impairments to lesions in an area of left prefrontal cortex—later known as Broca's area—rejuvenated the project of localizing control of specific behaviors or mental abilities in particular regions of the brain. This was opposed by Wernicke (1874), who focused instead on connections between primary sensory and motor areas in explaining normal and pathological conditions. But even proponents of this associationist approach, such as Hughlings Jackson (1884), spoke of the brain as representing and re-representing features of the world.

Localizationist research gave rise to the positing of representations in the brain as researchers began to identify specific brain regions responsible for particular kinds of sensory processing or motor control. Vision researchers, for example, initially simply sought the locus where visual

---

[2]Vogeley and Bartels in Chapter 8 of this volume advocate a functional role account of representation, contending that it best fits the practice of cognitive neuroscience research. I would argue that a functional role account is not an alternative to the control theoretic framework I offer here, or even to accounts that emphasize just the causal processes generating representations or their consumption, but rather is appropriate in analyzing control systems, such as cognitive systems, in which multiple representations are deployed in complex relations to each other so as to regulate the plant. In such situations a major task in the analysis is to understand how the various representations relate to each other. However, if the whole system of representations is not grounded in causal connections to what is represented and is not employed in regulating behavior, then it is not clear why the different roles within a system serve a representational function.

information was processed in the brain. Relying on both lesion studies and electrical stimulation, Ferrier (1876) argued for a locus in the angular gyrus, whereas Munk (1881) defended a locus in the occipital lobe that had earlier been distinguished by its pattern of striation and would later be known as the striate cortex. A variety of investigatory strategies soon settled the issue in favor of striate cortex. As techniques were refined, though, researchers began to investigate which parts of striate cortex responded to which parts of the visual field, treating it as embodying a map of the visual field. Henschen (1893) offered the first account of such a map, although ironically his proposal reversed the pattern of projection supported in subsequent research by Inouye (1909) and Holmes (1918).

The characterization of areas of cortex as possessing a map of the visual world clearly adopts a representational perspective, and the quest to specify maps became a major pursuit of neuroscientists in the 20th century. With the development of single cell recording techniques, investigators such as Talbot and Marshall (1941) began to focus on individual neurons. Following a strategy used in the retina and LGN by Kuffler (1953), Hubel and Wiesel (1962, 1968) investigated what features of a sensory stimulus would drive cells in striate cortex. Their discovery that simple visual features (oriented lines, stationary or moving in a particular direction) would elicit responses from specific cells in striate cortex, and that cells that responded to different features of a given stimulus were organized together within a column, led them to propose that information represented in one set of cells was further processed in others:

> We may tentatively look upon each column as a functional unit of cortex, within which simple fields are elaborated and then in turn synthesized into complex fields. The large variety of simple and complex fields to be found in a single column suggests that the connexions between cells in a column are highly specific (Hubel and Wiesel 1962, 144)

They also observed that this processing of oriented lines is "a very elementary stage in the handling of complex forms" and identified as a question for the future "how this information is used at later stages in the visual path" (Hubel and Wiesel 1968, 242).

Hubel, Wiesel, and others soon discovered that these later stages involved additional maps in occipital, temporal, and parietal cortex. Combining information from earlier stages in different ways, neurons in these areas analyzed visual stimuli in terms of such features as color, shape, direction of motion, and identity of objects (see Bechtel 2008, for details of this history). A similar history led to the identification of motor (Leyton and Sherrington 1917) and somatosensory (Penfield and Boldrey 1937) maps as well as tonotopic maps in auditory processing areas (Woolsey and Walzl 1942).[3] The advent of tools such as fMRI later fostered the discovery of maps in more anterior brain areas, notably those involved in attentional and working memory tasks (Sereno 2001, Hagler and Sereno 2006).

In this section I have described how neuroscientists seek to identify representations, especially maps, in the brain. Typically they do not elaborate on foundational issues, such as what it means to be a representation, what kinds of neural data license what kinds of inferences regarding representations, and the implications of these inferences and of representation talk more generally. Despite their reticence, it is fairly clear that the neuroscientists' approach is guided by the assumption Dretske articulated, according to which a process is presumed to carry information about its causes. Thus, techniques such as single cell recording and fMRI proceed by presenting stimuli (experimenter-designed causes) to the organism and recording the resulting activity in the brain. Neural maps are inferred from the correspondences found between the topology of the sensory field and that in the resulting map. Seldom as explicit as in Hubel and Wiesel's papers, but sometimes implicit, is a thorough-going analysis of how certain downstream brain areas act as consumers of these maps, typically by deriving from them more specialized maps, but sometimes instead using them to determine behavioral responses. In one of the most impressive studies pinning down a representational function in the brain, Britten et al. (1992) established the role of MT in representing motion by combining three kinds of data: (a) deficits in perceiving motion after lesions to MT; (b) single cell recording from MT during the presentation of motion stimuli; and (c) microstimulation of MT designed to bias a monkey's response to perceiving ambiguous motion displays. In their single-cell recording experiments the researchers were relying on the causal relation to the stimulus, while in appealing to the monkey's perceptual responses the researchers were targeting the consumer of this information.

---

[3] As in the case of vision, the discovery of one map was soon followed by additional maps. A second somatosensory map was identified by Woolsey (1943), and multiple auditory areas were discovered by Merzenich and Brugge (1973).

7.3 Dynamicists' Objections to Representations and the Control Theory Framework

Beginning in the 1990s, theorists advocating dynamical systems accounts of cognitive activity have challenged cognitive scientists' and neuroscientists' practice of ascribing mental representations. Sometimes their criticisms have focused on representations involving specific types of vehicles, notably the language-like representations employed in symbolic theories. But often the critics have targeted anything that might be construed as a representation. Van Gelder addressed his challenge to

> [...] pretty much any reasonable characterization, based around a core idea of some state of a system which, by virtue of some general representational scheme, stands in for some further state of affairs, thereby enabling the system to behave appropriately with respect to that state of affairs. (van Gelder 1995, 351)

The maps advanced by neuroscientists clearly fall within the scope of his challenge. To point the way towards accounting for cognition without appealing to representations, van Gelder presented the centrifugal governor that James Watt devised for the steam engine, which van Gelder maintains is "preferable to the Turing machine as a landmark for models of cognition" (van Gelder 1995, 381).

The governor is designed to regulate the flow of steam powering an engine such that the engine maintains as constant a speed as possible despite intermittent variability in load (e.g., from commercial sewing machines driven by the engine). Its key components are a spindle and two attached arms, each hinged with a heavy ball at the end. Figure 1 on the next page shows how one end of the governor is linked to the throttle valve used to modulate the supply of steam to the engine cylinder and the other end is directly connected to a flywheel or equivalent device. (This vintage diagram omits the rest of the engine, including the cylinder, the piston, and the output shaft and belt that drive the flywheel. Absent this primary mechanism, there would be nothing for the governor to govern.) At each moment the current engine speed is translated via the flywheel to the spindle and its attached arms. When the engine and hence the spindle speed up, centrifugal force drives the balls outwards, which increases the angle of the spindle arms, which lowers the arm of the linkage mechanism, which is attached to the valve in such a way that it partly closes. With less steam being supplied, the engine slows down. Conversely, when the engine slows down (due to this regulatory effect, fluctuations in the supply of steam, increased resistance in the machinery, etc.) there is less centrifugal force.

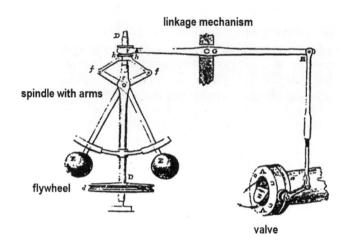

FIGURE 1   Watt's governor for the steam engine.
The figure is adapted from Farley (1827).

This lowers the balls, which decreases the angle of the spindle arms, which raises the linkage arm, which partly opens the valve, which increases the flow of steam, which speeds up the engine. There is, thus, a tight feedback loop that regulates the primary operation (steam-driven engine activity) with only a slight time lag.[4]

Van Gelder contended that the governor operates without representations and can be taken as a simple model for how a cognitive system could likewise function without representations. He offered several arguments for rejecting as "misleading"

> [...] a common and initially quite attractive intuition to the effect that the angle at which the arms are swinging is a representation of the current speed of the engine, and it is because the arms are related in this way to engine speed that the governor is able to control that speed (van Gelder 1995, 351).

Here I will consider just the first of these arguments, as doing so will help show why the "quite attractive intuition" is in fact correct (I have addressed his other arguments in Bechtel (1998)). In this argument van Gelder contended that there is no explanatory utility in construing the angle of the arms in representational terms; rather, a pair of differen-

---

[4]For a very illuminating discussion of the Watt governor, including its history and how, in some uses, it produces problematic oscillations, and the strategies engineers employed to cope with these, see Denny (2002).

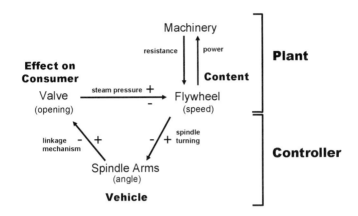

FIGURE 2 Schematic diagram showing how a representational system
(vehicle linked to content and consumer) is realized in the
control system architecture.

tial equations suffice to account for the operation of the governor: one
relating the acceleration in the angle of the arms to the engine speed
and current angle (see Equation (1) on page 139) and another relating
the engine speed to the angle of the arms. To answer van Gelder I will
argue that (a) a mechanistic analysis of the behavior of the governor
is informative and dovetails with the dynamical analysis and (b) that
mechanistic analysis of the governor requires a representational account
of the arm angles: they *stand in for* the speed of the engine and can
effectively regulate the valve opening *because* they do so.

A mechanistic analysis identifies parts of a system and the operations they perform, and shows how they are organized so as to generate
the phenomenon to be explained (Bechtel and Abrahamsen 2005). The
parts of this governor include the flywheel, spindle arms, and the linkage mechanism connected to the valve. As shown in Figure 2, each
component operates on a different engineering principle and hence performs a specific operation that contributes to the ability of the governor
to keep the engine operating at a constant speed. This exemplifies the
tasks in a mechanistic analysis: specifying each part and its operation
and connecting each operation to the functioning of the whole system.
The diagram makes it clear *why* Watt inserted the spindle arms: it
is *because* the spindle arms rise and fall in response to the speed of
the flywheel (and the engine more generally) and their angle can be
used by the linkage mechanism such that the valve will open and close

appropriately. Without the spindle arms and the appropriate linkage mechanism, the valve has no access to information about engine speed. Watt included them in the governor to encode that information in a format that the valve-opening mechanism could employ. This analysis illustrates a general point about representations: someone (a designer or evolution) has gone to the trouble of representing a state of affairs in a particular vehicle because that vehicle is suited for use by the consumer of that information.

While accepting the potential legitimacy of appeals to representation within this explanatory framework, Chemero (2000) challenged whether they do sufficient work.[5] In particular, he contended that when it comes to explaining how the Watt governor actually operates to regulate the behavior of the steam engine, one turns not to an account of its representational content, but to the dynamical equations that characterize its operations. To answer this objection, it is necessary to show how the dynamical equations that describe the Watt governor actually describe the representational content that the representational vehicles, the angle arms, provide to the consumer, the throttle valve, which then uses that content to appropriately adjust itself.[6] Nielsen (2010) shows that this is the case.

Nielsen's analysis starts with one of the two differential equations presented by van Gelder as jointly characterizing the operation of the governor, and which Chemoro argued provided a sufficient explanation of how the governor works. This equation, on its own, specifies the acceleration of the angle of the arms at time t given a particular engine speed:

---

[5]Chemero (2000) offered the following formal characterization of the role for representations, which agrees with the informal characterization I offered: "A feature R_0 of a system S will be counted as a Representation for S if and only if:

R1 R_0 stands between a representation producer P and a representation consumer C that have been standardized to fit one another.

R2 R_0 has as its proper function to adapt the representation consumer C to some aspect A_0 of the environment, in particular by leading S to behave appropriately with respect to A_0, even when A_0 is not the case.

R3 There are (in addition to R_0) transformations of $R_0, R_1, \ldots, R_n$, that have as their function to adapt the representation consumer C to corresponding transformations of $A_0, A_1, \ldots, A_n$." (Chemero 2000, 627)

[6]One of van Gelder's objections to treating the Watt governor representationally was that at best the angle arms misrepresent the speed of the flywheel because they are always slightly lagging behind it. My strategy in Bechtel (1998) was to appeal to Millikan's contention that something can represent even if it rarely or even never covaries with what it represents. Nielsen provides a much better response—the claim that the angle arms misrepresent the velocity of the flywheel stems from focusing only on the angle φ, not on the dynamic behavior of the angle arms, which includes their rate of change and acceleration.

$$(1) \qquad \frac{d^2\varphi}{dt^2} = (n\omega)^2 \cos\varphi \sin\varphi - \frac{g}{l}\sin\varphi - r\frac{d\varphi}{dt}$$

In this equation φ is the angle of the arms; ω is engine speed; and n, g, l, and r are parameters reflecting the gearing, gravity, length of the arms, and friction at the hinges respectively. To change the focus to how engine speed is represented in the behavior of the arms, Nielsen solves for ω:

$$(2) \qquad \omega = \frac{\sqrt{\dfrac{\dfrac{d^2\varphi}{dt^2} + \dfrac{g}{l}\sin\varphi + r\dfrac{d\varphi}{dt}}{\cos\varphi \sin\varphi}}}{n}$$

This reveals that engine speed at any point in time, t, is precisely represented by appropriate parameters and three variables characterizing the behavior of the angle arms at time t: φ, the current angle, $d\varphi/dt$, the rate of change in the angle, and $d^2\varphi/dt^2$, its acceleration.

There are limitations to Nielsen's analysis, since it captures only how engine speed is represented at a moment. Without the coupling of Equation (1) with a second equation characterizing the effect of the governor on the engine speed, the dynamic relation between ω and φ is not incorporated. It nonetheless illustrates the strategy of dynamic mechanistic analysis (Bechtel and Abrahamsen in press), insofar as it establishes a correspondence between variables in dynamic equations and properties of parts and operations of a mechanism and thereby coordinates what are often separate types of accounts into an especially revealing, integrated account. It also draws attention to an important aspect of the representational analysis of the Watt governor: in order to understand the representational content of the vehicle (the angle of the arms) it is necessary to view the vehicle dynamically—analyzing how the angle is changing—not just statically, as would be the case if only the current angle were considered. As Nielsen notes, the angle of the arms alone is ambiguous as the same angle will appear when the arms are rising and when they are falling, but in one case the valve will respond by closing to some degree whereas in the other it responds by opening to some degree. The velocity resolves this ambiguity: when the angle is increasing, the valve closes, whereas when it is decreasing, the valve opens.[7]

---

[7]The situation is far more complex when, as happened when steam engines became more powerful, the governor generates perpetual oscillations around the target value. In the original case Watt confronted, the oscillations were rapidly

Nielsen's analysis provides a compelling answer to Chemero's challenge; the dynamical analysis of the governor is in fact characterizing the representational content of the representational vehicle in the mechanism. But this response may fall victim to another objection to identifying representations in the Watt governor: the claim that characterizing a component of the mechanism as a representation is useful to the person trying to understand the operation of the mechanism, but that the mechanism itself has no actual representations (Haselager et al. 2003). The mechanism comprises only the parts and operations that produce its own behavior. To counter this objection it is fruitful to focus on what type of mechanism the Watt governor is. A governor or controller is that part of a mechanism (or submechanism, if it has multiple parts) that regulates the operation of other part(s)—i.e., one or more of those comprising the plant—by rendering them responsive to conditions internal or external to the plant. To regulate the plant the controller must be appropriately connected to it.[8] To make the plant responsive to conditions internal or external to it, the controller must carry information about them. This account of the controller turns out to employ precisely the two relations I previously described as crucial to representations. In the Watt governor, the changing angle of the arms is the vehicle and that vehicle is related both to the content of the representation (engine speed) and the consumer of the representation (the throttle valve). In general, if it were not for these two relations, controllers would not have been designed by engineers for machines and would not have evolved in organisms.

This suggests the hypothesis that the locus of representations is within control systems, and hence that representation cannot be understood apart from an understanding of control systems. Moreover, gaining such understanding involves exploration not only of the mechanical control systems conceived by engineers but also the far more ancient and widespread control systems in the biological world. The prevalence and importance of biological control systems can be recognized by considering the basic conditions in which organisms live.

---

dampened when perturbed only slightly from equilibrium, and so the focus of the analysis is on the equilibrium values.

[8]During many stages in its operation, representations in the controller may be detached from the current state of the plant. Many controllers use emulators to represent the plant when information from the plant is not directly available (Grush 2004). The circadian oscillator presented below in fact is often detached from the environmental cues that could inform it about time of day. However, if there is never an active coupling by which the operations in the governor are affected by operations in the plant, then the governor should not be credited with representing the plant.

They are systems far from thermodynamic equilibrium with their environment and must, if they are to maintain their identity, recruit matter and energy from their environment and deploy it to build and repair themselves (Ruiz-Mirazo et al. 2004). A basic component of all living systems is a boundary membrane, a semi-permeable boundary whose permeability can be modulated by the organism itself. Organisms also require operations for extracting energy from the materials that cross the membrane into the organism and utilization of this energy and matter to synthesize new parts, including the boundary membrane.[9] Continuous building and repair are essential operations in living mechanisms, as they must counter the basic tendency toward equilibrium exhibited by any system that is out of equilibrium with its environment (i.e., toward increased *entropy*—a general tendency throughout the physical world, including but not limited to organisms). It is conceivable that an organism could exist in which these ongoing operations are all adequately coupled to each other, such that it could survive and reproduce without any specialized regulatory system modulating and coordinating their dynamics. But such a mechanism would be extremely vulnerable, as it would be dependent upon its environment for provision of exactly the matter and energy it requires and for removal of its waste products precisely when necessary.

All known organisms, except perhaps for sulfur bacteria, must cope with variable environmental conditions and for this reason need to be flexible in deploying their component mechanisms. They therefore include control systems that serve to up- or down-regulate specific operations within the organism and to couple different operations so that they can be deployed in a coordinated manner. Such control need not be centralized and often involves signaling pathways through which the detection of internal or external circumstances directly triggers or shuts down the performance of an operation. Chemical signaling is common in single-celled organisms; in multi-celled organisms it is supplemented by neurons—cells specialized for faster and more directed communication via action potentials down axons. With the evolution of central ganglia and later of brains, ever more complex control systems appeared.

Control systems constitute the natural locus for representations, and the task of a control system is to acquire information that affects the plant being controlled and employ the information to regulate the

---

[9]Metabolism and construction of a membrane are two components of Gánti's (2003) conception of a chemoton, the simplest hypothetical physical system he could conceive that would exhibit the basic features of life. The third component is a control system, which he proposed could take the form of a component for constructing polymers whose length could then regulate other functions.

plant. Even the control systems employed in chemotaxis in bacteria are quite complex, involving parallel enzyme-mediated reactions, and to understand these it is necessary to focus on the information individual reactions are carrying and how the reaction pathways are linked. This is even more true when, in the cortex of mammals, multiple specialized brain areas process representations with different but related contents. The individual areas involve highly connected neurons that perform particular information processing operations, but these also need to be coordinated, which is achieved through a few long-range connections between areas dominated by local connections (Strogatz 2001, van Leeuwen 2007).

In the following section I will focus on one fundamental representational activity that, as far as we can tell, figures in the regulation of behavior of most organisms, namely, the representation of time and length of day. Before turning to that, though, I summarize the lessons I draw from reconsidering van Gelder's arguments. First, the introduction of the Watt governor as a kind of prototype for the design of cognitive systems was a happy choice. We should view the mind/brain as a controller (or, better, a collection of controllers) regulating an already active biological system. Accordingly, we should employ tools and perspectives from control theory in characterizing the design and functioning of the mind/brain. Second, as van Gelder suggested, the activities of the mind/brain may best be described in differential equations. Further, the tools of dynamical systems theory and complexity theory may generate some of the most informative accounts of the functioning of the mind/brain as a control system. But, third, doing so does not entail rejecting the characterization of brain activity in representational terms. Indeed, it is only by identifying their representational vehicles and understanding the content they carry that we understand how brains function as control systems. In pursuing this inquiry, our understanding of what representations are and how they are employed may radically change. One such change has already been noted: that it may be important to focus not on representational states but representational processes since some of the crucial information involves not the instantaneous state of a system but rather rates of change or acceleration of operations in that system.

7.4 A Dynamical System for Representing Time of Day

A wide range of physiological and behavioral activities of organisms are linked to particular periods of earth's 24-hour day: fruit flies eclose from pupae at dawn (Pittendrigh 1960–1961), cyanobacteria fix nitrogen at night (Golden et al. 1997), chipmunks forage at times best suited to avoid predators (DeCoursey et al. 2000), and humans exhibit their quickest reaction times shortly after midday. In these and numerous other cases, physiological and behavioral activities remain keyed to time of day even in the absence of all external cues such as daylight or temperature changes. That is, the timing of activities is under substantial endogenous control: organisms represent time of day through some internal process and use it to regulate their activities. One of the clearest examples is that animal species (both invertebrate and vertebrate) have preferred times to sleep. Even if an animal is deprived of sleep during this period and thereby suffers a sleep deficit, it will tend to delay its subsequent sleep to the preferred time.[10]

Researchers commonly refer to the mechanism responsible for daily timekeeping as a *clock*. Since, in the absence of external cues, most organisms maintain a highly reliable cycle with a period of approximately but not exactly 24 hours, it is called a *circadian* (*circa* = about + *dies* = day) clock. The assumption that there exists *a* clock reflects a common research heuristic: when a system performs some activity, assume one part of the system is responsible for it. This assumption, which Richardson and I (Bechtel and Richardson 1993) labeled *direct* or *simple localization*, is fallible in that the activity may actually result from the coordinated operation of many components, not just (or even including) the one initially identified. Even though there are now good reasons to challenge the assumption of a single clock,[11] it paid off handsomely in animal research as researchers were able to localize the presumed clock in particular parts of organisms' brains. In mammals

---

[10]Time periods for sleep are regulated independently from the amount of sleep required. Organisms deprived of sleep will compensate with increased intensity and duration in subsequent sleep episodes, a phenomenon known as sleep homeostasis (Saper et al. 2005).

[11]Typically, across many fields of science, when a direct localization is hypothesized it turns out to be correct only to a first approximation. In the case of circadian timekeeping, the same basic mechanism is present in many cells distributed through the animal's body. These cells maintain oscillations, but fail to synchronize without input from the SCN. Within the SCN individual cells vary considerably in their periodicity so that the regular oscillatory pattern exhibited in behavior depends upon the integration of individual cells' behavior into stable collective behavior via intra-SCN synchronization.

this was the suprachiasmatic nucleus (SCN) of the hypothalamus, a structure residing just above the optic chiasm where the nerve projections from the two eyes come together before resegregating *en route* to the thalamus. Several lines of evidence support the claim that the SCN is the central clock: lesioning the SCN renders mammals arrhythmic (Moore and Eichler 1972), transplanting a donor SCN into animals whose own SCN has been removed restores rhythmic behavior (Ralph et al. 1990), and many neurons in SCN explants maintained in culture generate circadian rhythms (Welsh et al. 1995).

The SCN indeed is the mammalian central clock, but this direct localization was only the first step towards a far more complex account. A key part of the mechanism is in fact molecular and intracellular: its primary parts and operations have been identified and are now known to be replicated not only within individual neurons in the SCN but also, as peripheral clocks, in somatic cells of the liver and other organs. The first clue towards a molecular decomposition of the central clock came from research on fruit flies (*Drosophila*) in which Konopka and Benzer (1971) succeeded in generating mutants that exhibited shortened or lengthened circadian rhythms or became arrhythmic. They named the gene that had been altered to produce these effects *period* (*per*). The development of cloning techniques in the 1980s enabled Rosbash and his collaborators to identify *per*'s mRNA transcript and the resulting protein, PER. Hardin et al. (1990) established that concentrations of both *per* mRNA and PER exhibited circadian rhythms, with the peaks and valleys in PER concentration following those of *per* mRNA by about eight hours. Further, they determined that these oscillations were shortened, lengthened, or absent in mutants of the types first generated by Konopka and Benzer. Based on these results, Hardin et al. (1990) proposed a feedback mechanism in which, once PER has been synthesized in the cytoplasm, it is transported back into the nucleus where, in some way not understood at the time, it inhibits expression of the gene *per* and hence its own further synthesis (cf. Figure 3 on the next page). Assuming this account of the mechanism (it later turned out to be more complex), here is an intuitive understanding of how it would generate oscillations. When concentrations of PER in the nucleus are low, gene expression proceeds normally, leading to a gradual buildup of PER in the cytoplasm towards its peak concentration there. This buildup would be countered by breakdown over time of PER molecules; some, however, are first transported into the nucleus, where their concentration peaks approximately 8 hours after that of *per* mRNA. This inhibits further transcription of *per*, which leads to a gradual reduction of PER in the cytoplasm. But on this account, another operation also

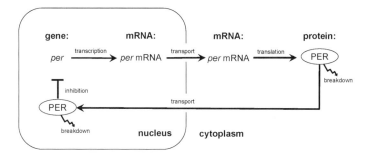

FIGURE 3 Hardin's (1990) proposed feedback mechanism
for generating circadian oscillations in fruit flies.

plays a role in producing oscillations in concentrations: as in the cytoplasm, the PER molecules in the nucleus break down over time. As its
nuclear concentration declined, PER's inhibitory effect on *per* declines
as well. Consequently, transcription and translation gradually return
to their maximum rate, and PER levels in the cytoplasm recover. This
negative feedback loop would repeat indefinitely; and assuming that
the various operations proceed at appropriate rates, the resulting oscillations in concentrations of the molecules can be envisaged as taking
approximately 24 hours.[12]

Arriving at this proposed mechanistic explanation drew on the
strategies common to most biological research: *simple localization* of
the overall mechanism (for mammals, in the SCN); *decomposition* of
that mechanism into its parts (*per, per* mRNA, PER) and their operations (transcription, transport, translation, inhibition, and breakdown);
and *recomposition* of the component parts and operations into a complex mechanism capable of producing the phenomenon of interest (see
Bechtel and Abrahamsen 2009). As the first such proposal it was a
landmark that guided future research; but as one would expect, it was
incomplete in numerous respects. The ensuing two decades of research
have yielded a much more complete mechanistic account of circadian
clocks. One gap was recognized almost immediately—since PER has no
DNA binding region, PER molecules could not directly act on the *per*
gene to inhibit transcription of additional PER molecules. Following

---

[12]Such intuitive reasoning is fallible. The initial oscillations in such a mechanism
potentially could dampen as the concentrations approach a steady state. To show
that such a mechanism would in fact sustain oscillations requires mathematical modeling; Goldbeter (1995b) developed such a model and, using biologically plausible
parameter values, achieved oscillatory behavior.

the same research strategy that had successfully identified *per* in fruit flies, Vitaterna et al. (1994) sought and found in mice a gene that they named *Clock* (for *circadian locomotor output cycles kaput*). When the mutant gene was heterozygous, it resulted in a lengthened period; when homozygous, it resulted in loss of circadian rhythms within two weeks. When the group succeeded in cloning *Clock* two years later, they correctly predicted "that this candidate gene encodes a novel member of the bHLH-PAS domain family of transcription factors" (King et al. 1997, 645). Such a transcription factor would enable binding to a site known as an E-box on the promoter of another gene such as *per*. Shortly thereafter Darlington et al. (1998) found a homolog of *Clock* in fruit flies and, conversely, Sun et al. (1997) demonstrated the existence of a mammalian homolog of *per*. This established a basic parallel between the clock mechanisms of fruit flies and mammals. (There were also many differences of detail; for example, it was soon found that mammals have three homologues to *per*, at least two of which (*mPer1* and *mPer2*) code for clock proteins.) In fruit flies, Gekakis et al. (1998) hypothesized that PER in some way alters the ability of CLOCK to bind with the E-box on the *per* promoter. Other research in the 1990s and beyond revealed additional complexities in the clock mechanism. There were corresponding findings for fruit flies, but focusing here just on mammals, it was found that both proteins function by forming dimers (compounds) with other proteins (PER with CRY and CLOCK with BMAL1). Another complexity is the discovery of a second, positive feedback loop in which the dimer formed by CLOCK and BMAL1 also binds to the E-Box on the promoter of RORα, which in turn binds to the RORE-box on the promoter of BMAL1, so that BMAL1 stimulates production of more of itself. Figure 4 on the facing page shows the current conception of the organization of the mammalian clock mechanism.

I have focused on how molecular operations within individual SCN generate a 24-hour oscillation in concentrations of mRNA transcripts and proteins. In the next section I will address how these operations carry information about time of day and are used by the organism because they do so, thereby establishing that they represent time of day. Before doing so, though, I should note that while uncovering this intracellular mechanism was absolutely crucial, investigations targeting a higher level of organization have helped flesh out how 24-hour oscillations are maintained (for further discussion, see Bechtel and Abrahamsen 2009). These investigations, with an intercellular rather than intracellular focus, examined the SCN as a network of neurons that could influence one another's behavior. Consider what happened when

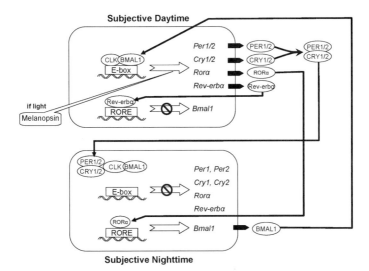

FIGURE 4 The basic components of the mammalian circadian oscillator.
During subjective day, the CLK:BMAL1 dimer binds to the E-box promoter
on the *Per1*, *Per2*, *Cry1*, *Cry2*, *RORα* and *Rev-erbα* genes, activating
expression of these genes. During subjective night, the PER:CRY dimers
interact with the CLK:BMAL1 dimers, removing them from the E-boxes
and hence inhibiting gene expression. The *Bmal1* gene has the opposite
cycle, inhibited during subjective day but activated during subjective night.
The large open arrows indicate whether gene expression is activated or
inhibited. The smaller filled arrows represent the combined operations of
gene expression that are shown individually in Figure 3 on page 145
(transcription, transport, and translation into the appropriate protein).

Welsh et al. (1995) dispersed neurons from the SCN of mice on multi-
electrode grids. They produced the first demonstration that individual
SCN cells exhibit regular oscillations in their rates of neural activity. But they also noted an important unexpected finding: considerable
variability across cells in their period of oscillation, ranging from 21.25
hours to 26.25 hours with a SD of 1.25 hours. This was in stark contrast to the low variability exhibited by whole organisms on behavioral
measures; for example, individual mice are very regular in the time of
day at which they attain peaks in their wheel running and other activities. Moreover, when Herzog et al. (2004) maintained the pattern
of neural connectivity in slices they found much less variability. This
suggested that oscillations in neural activity somehow become synchronized when neurons are organized into a network within the SCN. The

same laboratory soon produced evidence pointing to vasoactive intestinal peptide (VIP) as the synchronizing agent, and considerable research subsequently has been devoted to the process and pattern of synchronization (Welsh et al. 2010). Other research has established that even when the period of increased activity is well-synchronized across neurons in SGN, individual neurons differ in the time at which activity peaks; also, these times are more widely dispersed on days with longer photoperiods than on days with shorter photoperiods (Schaap et al. 2003, van der Leest et al. 2007). The result is that on days with short photoperiods, the amplitude of the waveform generated by electrical activity over the whole SCN is greater, providing a possible encoding of photoperiod that could be used to regulate activities that must be performed on shorter or longer days over the course of the year.

7.5 Responding to Referents and Informing Consumers

In the previous section I sketched the research that in the past two decades has revealed the mechanisms which endogenously generate circadian oscillations within SCN cells—as revealed in both gene expression and electrical activity—and synchronize oscillations between SCN cells as well. This does not yet establish that these oscillations satisfy the control-theoretic account of representation I presented in Section 7.3. Many other oscillatory processes have been found in organisms, some of which perform important regulatory functions while others apparently do not (Goldbeter 1995a, Buzsáki 2006). Because most do not carry information about external cyclic phenomena, there is no compelling reason to think of them as representing temporal processes outside themselves. In order to show, on the control-theory account, that circadian oscillations in the SCN constitutes a clock—that they represent time of day—they must be shown to carry information about time of day (the referent of the representation). Further, the fact that they carry information about time of day must figure in how the activity in the SCN is consumed. The activities elsewhere in the organism that are affected by the oscillations in the SCN must be ones that need information about time of day to be performed effectively.

Considerable progress has been made in identifying the processes by which the SCN oscillations are normally linked to actual time of day, although they can be maintained even under constant conditions in which they receive no information about time of day. There are several sources of information from which an organism can gain information about time of day—light, ambient temperature, food availability, and physical activity all are effective under appropriate circumstances—but the onset and offset of daylight is the most effective source for entraining circadian oscillators. In mammals there is a direct neural pathway—the hypothalamic tract—from the retina of the eye to the SCN. It was the discovery of this pathway that initially led Moore and Eichler (1972)[13] to focus on the SCN as a candidate locus for the clock. At the molecular level, almost immediately after the discovery of the mammalian homologues of *per*, Shigeyoshi et al. (1997) determined that exposure to light induced expression of *mPer1* in SCN cells; subsequent research showed that *mPer2* was similarly affected, but not *mPer3* (Zylka et al. 1998). This research established that light exposure has causal effects in the SCN, but did not reveal the mediating mechanism. The determination that organisms in which rods and cones are destroyed can still entrain to light, while those without eyes cannot, pointed to the existence of an additional type of photosensitive cell in the eye. Working with the frog *Xenopus laevis*, Provencio et al. (1998) discovered a new member of the opsin family, melanopsin, in melanophores (melanin pigment containing cells). Subsequently they determined that melanopsin is present in the mammalian inner retina (Provencio et al. 2002), which helped resolve the puzzle and established melanopsin at the input end of the pathway.[14]

The task was then to fill in the intermediate steps by which information about light is transmitted to the SCN. Crosio et al. (2000) showed that increased transcription of *mPer1* and *mPer2* resulted from chromatin remodeling (a process that alters the manner in which DNA wraps around histones and thereby affects whether the enzymes required for transcription can attach to the DNA). Soon thereafter Travnickova-Bendova et al. (2002) offered evidence that the final pathway involves a cAMP response element (CRE) phosphorylating a CRE-binding protein (CREB), which binds to promoter sites on *mPer1* and *mPer2* to initiate transcription. A role was also established for PACAP (*pituitary adenylate cyclase activating peptide*), a neurotransmitter active in the retinohypothalamic tract during subjective day. At the input

---

[13]Moore was initially searching for the visual pathway that controlled pineal biosynthetic activities.

[14]The discovery that mice mutants lacking melanopsin can still entrain to bright light, albeit with less responsiveness than wild types to pulses of light, indicated that the dismissal of rods and cones as playing a role in entrainment had been premature (Panda et al. 2003, Hattar et al. 2003). Dkhissi-Benyahya et al. (2007) demonstrated that a mid-wavelength opsin (peak sensitivity above 530 nm) found in cones was the likely agent of entrainment via cones. Hatori et al. (2008) showed that the entrainment produced from the cones is mediated by the melanopsin-expressing retinal ganglion cells.

end, Hannibal et al. (2002) established that in mammals melanopsin is found in the same inner retinal ganglion cells as PACAP. Moreover, PACAP receptors were identified on SCN cells, and a signaling pathway within SCN neurons was proposed whereby PACAP binding initiates the sequence culminating in CRE phosphorylating CREB. Thus, in less than five years researchers had identified the main components and achieved a coherent account of how light entrains the mammalian clock.[15] This establishes that the circadian oscillations of PER and other clock proteins in the SCN cells carry information about time of day since they are typically entrained to the day-night cycle on the planet (the referent). The fact that entrainment only occurs at certain times of day and that when entrainment is impaired, oscillations continue, does not jeopardize the claim that the content of the representation is time of day, for that is what the consumer components of the organism (the plant) require information about in order to time their own operations in order for them to be effective.

Turning to the consumer side, there is overwhelming evidence that oscillations in protein concentrations within the SCN are used to coordinate the timing of various mammalian activities, although many of the details of how they do so remain obscure. Part of the challenge is the extraordinary range of physiological and behavioral activities that exhibit circadian regulation. These include sleep, cardiovascular activity, endocrine levels, body temperature, renal activity, gastro-intestinal tract activity, hepatic metabolism, and motor activities. These various activities all exhibit circadian oscillations, but differ in the time at which they initiate and peak. Accordingly, they differ in the way they utilize the SCN oscillator in controlling these activities.

The mechanisms involved in many of these activities are not well understood, making it difficult to establish the detailed connections between the protein oscillations in SCN cells and the regulation of these activities. It is, however, clear that circadian oscillations in these activities are regulated by the SCN. The pioneering studies identifying the SCN as the locus of the central clock showed that lesions to the SCN in rats eliminated circadian control of adrenal corticosterone (Moore and Eichler 1972) and of drinking and locomotion (Stephan and Zucker

---

[15] A further aspect of entrainment is that light is effective in resetting the circadian oscillator only during the night, and it is most effective immediately after subjective dusk and before subjective dawn. Light delivered during the middle of the subjective night can so disrupt circadian oscillations as to render the organism arrhythmic, an effect first hypothesized by Winfree (1970) and confirmed in subsequent research (Honma and Honma 1999). Research on the mechanism has now suggested why light at different times is responded to differently (Pulivarthy et al. 2007).

1972). Transplant studies in the 1980s on lesioned rats that had been rendered arrhythmic established that transplanting SCN tissue from intact rats into the third ventricle could restore circadian motor activity, but not endocrine oscillations (Drucker-Colin et al. 1984, Sawaki et al. 1984, Lehman et al. 1987). If the donor tissue is from a mutant with a different circadian period, circadian behavior in the host will reflect that of the donor (Ralph et al. 1990).

These lesion and transplant studies provide compelling evidence that oscillations in the SCN are used elsewhere in the body as a source of information about time of day so as to coordinate behaviors. A clue to how this is accomplished emerged along with the discovery of mammalian clock genes *Clock* and *mPer1* and *mPer2*, as they were found to cycle not just in the SCN but in organs throughout the body (King et al. 1997, Sun et al. 1997).[16] Balsalobre et al. (1998) demonstrated that with serum shock they could induce circadian oscillations in rat fibroblast tissue kept in culture for more than 25 years and concluded:

> On the basis of our results with fibroblasts and hepatoma cells, it appears that peripheral tissues contain a clock capable of measuring time with impressive precision. One can thus hypothesize that many circadian outputs might be controlled by peripheral clocks, which may themselves be synchronized by the central clock (Balsalobre et al. 1998, 934).

Subsequently, peripheral clocks have been shown to regulate the rhythmic generation of numerous transcription factors such as *Dbp*, *Hlf*, and *Tef* (Gachon et al. 2006), and *E4bp4*, which oscillates out of phase with the others and competes for their binding sites on regulated genes (Mitsui et al. 2001). These transcription factors provide circadian regulation of clock controlled genes. Researchers have found that in any given tissue approximately 10% of genes exhibit a circadian pattern of expression, with the specific genes showing such a pattern varying by tissue type (Storch et al. 2002, Panda et al. 2002).

Peripheral clocks thus appear to play an important mediating role in the consumption of the SCN oscillations. The understanding of the way in which peripheral clocks are dependent on the SCN has under-

---

[16]Rhythmic expression of clock genes was first identified in fruit flies both in the central nervous system, especially the visual system, and in the digestive track (Siwicki et al. 1988). The development of techniques for fusing the luciferase gene *luc* to the *per* gene facilitated the creation of transgenic flies in which bioluminescence accompanies *per* expression. This enabled Plautz et al. (1997) to demonstrate *per* oscillations in dissociated head, thorax, and abdomen tissue from flies. With *per* driven green fluorescent protein (GFP) they found oscillations in the probiscus, antennae, legs, and wings. All these oscillators were able to entrain anew when the photoperiod was advanced or retarded.

gone major revision in recent years. When peripheral clocks were first identified in the late 1990s, it was assumed that they dampened after a few cycles of oscillation without inputs from the SCN (Yamazaki et al. 2000). This led researchers to view the SCN as the master clock and peripheral clocks as slaves (Akhtar et al. 2002). There had long been behavioral evidence, however, suggesting the existence of sustained circadian oscillators outside the SCN. Shortly after the discovery of the role of the SCN in most circadian behavior, several researchers determined that SCN lesioned rats that are fed at regular but restricted times anticipate their mealtime (Stephan et al. 1979). The fact that the food anticipatory behavior (locomotor activity and body temperature changes) free runs during periods of food deprivation and shows a transient effect as the organism adjusts to phase shifts in feeding times indicates that it is governed by a circadian clock distinct from that in the SCN (Davidson and Stephan 1999). Even with the SCN intact, gene expression in the liver, kidney, heart, and other tissues can be altered by changes in feeding time while leaving the phase of gene expression in the SCN unaffected (Damiola et al. 2000).[17]

Nonetheless, the assumption that peripheral clocks could not sustain oscillation unless they received input from the SCN or Zeitgebers (environmental time cues such as light) persisted until Yoo et al. (2004), using a luciferase reporter that enabled tracking oscillations of *per* transcription in individual cells, showed that liver and lung explants can maintain rhythmicity for at least 20 cycles. They concluded that the appearance of dampening was due to the fact that individual oscillators were no longer synchronized and so, at a population level, the oscillations in individual cells cancelled out. This prompted Davidson et al. (2004) to propose the orchestra conductor metaphor as preferable to the slave master metaphor:

> He [the conductor] uses a baton rather than a whip because musicians (peripheral oscillators) are independent interpreters in their own right and must be coaxed, not driven. The aesthetic quality of the performance (fitness) depends heavily on how successfully the flow of information (coupling) regulates synchrony among the performers (Davidson et al. 2004, 119).

---

[17]The effect of eating on the phase of the liver oscillator may be mediated by the increase in NAD^+ levels (levels are decreased in muscle and fat tissue), likely as a result of fat synthesis. The effect of NAD^+ on circadian oscillations may in part be direct, as the ratio of NADH to NAD^+ (or NADPH to $NADP^+$) can affect the binding of the CLOCK:BMAL1 or CLOCK:NPAS2 to DNA (Rutter et al. 2001). But there is also evidence that it is mediated by SIRT1 (Sirtuin 1), an NAD^+-dependent histone deacetylase that binds with CLOCK:BMAL1 and promotes the deacetylation and degradation of PER2 (Asher et al. 2008, Nakahata et al. 2008).

The conductor metaphor captures the representational perspective I am advancing here. Insofar as the SCN is the conductor, it is producing representations that peripheral clocks (orchestra players) employ in regulating physiological systems (their instruments). In the framework I have been developing, the conductor is the central controller, the orchestra players are controllers in peripheral systems, and the instruments are the plants that are regulated.

Evidence thus strongly suggests that the SCN's representation of time of day is consumed by peripheral oscillators and by this means their timekeeping is coordinated with that of the SCN. The details of how information is transmitted are not yet known, but some steps in the process have been identified. The SCN is itself divided into two major regions, the core and shell. The core sends projections to the shell and also to the lateral parasubventricular zone ($_L$SPV) of the hypothalamus, while the shell sends outputs to the paraventricular nucleus of the thalamus (PVT), the paraventricular nucleus of the hypothalamus (PVN), the medial subparaventricular zone ($_M$SPV), the preoptic area (POA), and the dorsomedial hypothalamic nucleus (DMH). These areas in turn send projections to many other regions of the body. However, the SCN is not solely dependent on neuronal output. In transplant experiments in hamsters, even when the donor SCN was encased in a semipermeable polymeric capsule and so developed no neuronal connections, the donor could promote rhythmic behavior (Silver et al. 1996). This suggests an important role for hormonal outputs from the SCN. Several peptides exhibit circadian oscillations and are thought likely to be regulated by central clock components: AVP (vasopressin), PK2 (prokineticin-2), TGFα (transforming growth factor-α), and a cardiotrophin-like cytokine (Antle and Silver 2005, Kalsbeek et al. 2006). TGFα inhibits locomotor activity by acting on receptors in the hypothalamic subparaventricular zone (SPZ), which also is a major relay station for SCN neuronal efferents (Kramer et al. 2001). PK2 also suppresses locomotor activity, but not by affecting the SPZ. There thus appear to be multiple pathways by which information from the SCN is transmitted to its various consumers. This is fitting given that the various consumers differ in the preferred time of day for their activities.

Existing accounts of how the SCN oscillators are entrained by light, how they orchestrate oscillations in peripheral oscillators, and how these oscillators can be entrained by Zeitgebers other than light are still incomplete, but there is little reason to be dubious that such connections exist. We can be confident that the SCN has appropriate connections to information about time of day and to consumers of such information, and hence can be credited with *representing* that information for mammals.

7.6 Conclusion: Representations as Components of Control Systems

The embrace of representations in the cognitive and neural sciences has been challenged by advocates of a contentiously narrow dynamical systems approach. In this paper I have pursued how a different stance—dynamic mechanistic explanation—can bring together the dynamical and representationalist perspectives rather than set them in opposition. I showed that even the Watt governor, which van Gelder advanced as a paradigm case of dynamics without representation, exemplifies this hybrid approach, by which representations invariably arise in the functioning of any dynamical system that incorporates a control system. Within this perspective I have explored both how dynamical processes within controllers carry information about the plant and its environment, and on how the plant consumes this information, but my main concern has been the implications of construing control systems themselves as the loci of representations. In particular, given a control system, one does not need to speculate further about how selection might have favored the representational system—it is sufficient to understand how representations arise within the controller and are used to coordinate behavior.

In suggesting that control systems provide a novel and informative framework in which to understand representations, I not only showed how representations arise in the Watt governor, but examined a biological case—the circadian clock that represents time and length of day. Circadian clocks utilize intracellular oscillatory processes to maintain an endogenous timing signal. In all but bacteria, the oscillation occurs when proteins synthesized from a few particular genes feed back in an inhibitory manner on that same process of gene expression. This internal oscillation is entrained by Zeitgebers such as light so as to align its phase with the day-night cycle in the world. Moreover, it is used in varying ways to regulate physiological and behavioral activities of the organism. From within a control theory perspective, the common objection to the notion of representation—that this is purely a convenience to theorists—gains little traction. A control system, such as the SCN, can regulate an organism's behavior only if it represents the relevant information about the plant (the rest of the organism's brain and body) and the conditions impinging on it and uses this information (dynamically varying representations) in directing the plant. If it does not encode the relevant information, the controller is unable to perform its function in the organism.

On the account I am advancing, representations have their home within, and are essential to, a particular type of mechanism—a control system. A simple feedback mechanism such as the Watt governor is the simplest exemplar. More elaborate mechanisms, such as the circadian clock, can represent dynamic information even when no current input from the referent is available (they are what Grush has characterized as emulators). Other neural and cognitive systems make more elaborate use of representations, and extending this basic account to these contexts in which more elaborate mechanisms are involved will require considerable additional work (see Barsalou 1999, for an account of concepts grounded in basic sensory motor processes that offers a promising route for doing so).[18] An advantage of having begun with a representational system which appears to be present in all five kingdoms of living organisms—the circadian clock—is that it compellingly illustrates that the challenge of linking representational vehicles to their content need not be daunting if we focus on the right kind of mechanism—a control system linked to a plant.

Acknowledgements

I thank an anonymous reviewer and Sebo Uithol as well as participants in the December 2008 workshop on the Concept of Representation in Neuroscience in Bonn, Germany, and audiences at the University of Bristol and University of Murcia for their helpful comments and suggestions.

References

Akhtar, R.A., A.B. Reddy, E.S. Maywood, J.D. Clayton, V.M. King, A.G. Smith, T.W. Gant, M.H. Hastings, and C.P. Kyriacou. 2002. Circadian cycling of the mouse liver transcriptome, as revealed by cDNA microarray, is driven by the suprachiasmatic nucleus. *Current Biology* 12 (7):540–550.

Antle, M.C. and R. Silver. 2005. Orchestrating time: arrangements of the brain circadian clock. *Trends in Neurosciences* 28 (3):145–151.

Asher, G., D. Gatfield, M. Stratmann, H. Reinke, C. Dibner, F. Kreppel, R. Mostoslavsky, F.W. Alt, and U. Schibler. 2008. SIRT1 regulates circa-

---

[18]In cognitive control systems multiple representations are processed in the same system, and a major challenge in understanding such systems is to understand how these representations relate to one another. In this context, focusing on the functional role of representations, as discussed in Vogeley and Bartels' paper in Chapter 8 of this volume, is critical. As discussed in note 2 on page 132 above, this is not incompatible with the control theoretical perspective advanced here.

dian clock gene expression through PER2 deacetylation. *Cell* 134 (2):317–328.

Balsalobre, A., F. Damiola, and U. Schibler. 1998. A serum shock induces circadian gene expression in mammalian tissue culture cells. *Cell* 93 (6):929–937.

Barsalou, L.W. 1999. Perceptual symbol systems. *Behavioral and Brain Sciences* 22:577–660.

Bechtel, W. 1998. Representations and cognitive explanations: Assessing the dynamicist's challenge in cognitive science. *Cognitive Science* 22:295–318.

Bechtel, W. 2008. *Mental mechanisms*. Routledge.

Bechtel, W. and A. Abrahamsen. 2005. Explanation: A mechanist alternative. *Studies in History and Philosophy of Biological and Biomedical Sciences* 36:421–441.

Bechtel, W. and A. Abrahamsen. 2009. Decomposing, recomposing, and situating circadian mechanisms: Three tasks in developing mechanistic explanations. In H. Leitgeb and A. Hieke, eds., *Reduction and elimination in philosophy of mind and philosophy of neuroscience*, pages 173–186. Ontos Verlag.

Bechtel, W. and A. Abrahamsen. in press. Complex biological mechanisms: Cyclic, oscillatory, and autonomous. In C. Hooker, ed., *Philosophy of complex systems. Handbook of the philosophy of science*, vol. 10. Elsevier.

Bechtel, W. and R.C. Richardson. 1993. *Discovering complexity: Decomposition and localization as strategies in scientific research*. Princeton University Press.

Brentano, F. 1874. *Psychology from an empirical standpoint*. Humanities.

Britten, K.H., M.N. Shadlen, W.T. Newsome, and J.A. Movshon. 1992. The analysis of visual motion: A comparison of neuronal and psychophysical performance. *Journal of Neuroscience* 12:4745–4765.

Broca, P. 1861. Remarques sur le siége de la faculté du langage articulé, suivies d'une observation d'aphemie (perte de la parole). *Bulletin de la Société Anatomique* 6:343–357.

Buzsáki, G. 2006. *Rhythms of the brain*. Oxford University Press.

Chemero, A. 2000. Anti-representationalism and the dynamical stance. *Philosophy of Science* 67 (4):625–647.

Crosio, C., N. Cermakian, C.D. Allis, and P. Sassone-Corsi. 2000. Light induces chromatin modification in cells of the mammalian circadian clock. *Nature Neuroscience* 3 (12):1241–1247.

Damiola, F., N. Le Minh, N. Preitner, B. Kornmann, F. Fleury-Olela, and U. Schibler. 2000. Restricted feeding uncouples circadian oscillators in peripheral tissues from the central pacemaker in the suprachiasmatic nucleus. *Genes and Development* 14 (23):2950–2961.

Darlington, T.K., K. Wager-Smith, M.F. Ceriani, D. Staknis, N. Gekakis, T.D. Steeves, N. Gekakis, C.J. Weitz, J.S. Takahashi, and S.A. Kay. 1998. Closing the circadian loop: CLOCK-induced transcription of its own inhibitors *per* and *tim*. *Science* 280 (5369):1599–1603.

Davidson, A.J. and F.K. Stephan. 1999. Feeding-entrained circadian rhythms in hypophysectomized rats with suprachiasmatic nucleus lesions. *American Journal of Physiology: Regulatory, Integrative, and Comparative Physiology* 277 (5):R1376–1384.

Davidson, A.J., S. Yamazaki, and M. Menaker. 2004. SCN: Ringmaster of the circadian circus or conductor of the circadian orchestra? In D. Chadwick and J. Goode, eds., *Molecular clocks and light signalling*, pages 110–125. John Wiley.

DeCoursey, P.J., J.K. Walker, and S.A. Smith. 2000. A circadian pacemaker in free-living chipmunks: essential for survival? *Journal of Comparative Physiology A: Neuroethology, Sensory, Neural, and Behavioral Physiology* 186 (2):169–180.

Denny, M. 2002. Watt steam governor stability. *European Journal of Physics* 23 (3):339–351.

Dkhissi-Benyahya, O., C. Gronfier, W. DeVanssay, F. Flamant, and H.M. Cooper. 2007. Modeling the role of mid-wavelength cones in circadian responses to light. *Neuron* 33 (5):677–687.

Dretske, F.I. 1981. *Knowledge and the flow of information.* MIT Press/Bradford Books.

Drucker-Colin, R., R. Aguilar-Roblero, F. Garcia-Hernandez, F. Fernandez-Cancino, and F.B. Rattoni. 1984. Fetal suprachiasmatic nucleus transplants: diurnal rhythm recovery of lesioned rats. *Brain Research* 311 (2):353–357.

Farley, J. 1827. *A treatise on the steam engine: Historical, practical, and descriptive.* Longman, Rees, Orme, Brown, and Green.

Ferrier, D. 1876. *The functions of the brain.* Smith, Elder, and Company.

Fodor, J.A. 1990. *A theory of content and other essays.* MIT Press.

Gachon, F., F.F. Olela, O. Schaad, P. Descombes, and U. Schibler. 2006. The circadian PAR-domain basic leucine zipper transcription factors DBP, TEF, and HLF modulate basal and inducible xenobiotic detoxification. *Cell Metabolism* 4 (1):25–36.

Gall, F.J. 1812. *Anatomie et physiologie du système nerveaux et général, et du cerveau en particulier, avec des observations sur la possibilité de reconnoitre plusieurs dispositions intellectuelles et morales de l'homme et des animaux, par la configuration de leur têtes.* F. Schoell.

Gánti, T. 2003. *The principles of life.* Oxford Univerity Press.

Gekakis, N., D. Staknis, H.B. Nguyen, F.C. Davis, L.D. Wilsbacher, D.P. King, J.S. Takahashi, and C.J. Weitz. 1998. Role of the CLOCK protein in the mammalian circadian mechanism. *Science* 280 (5369):1564–1569.

Goldbeter, A. 1995a. *Biochemical oscillations and cellular rhythms: The molecular bases of periodic and chaotic behaviour.* Cambridge University Press.

Goldbeter, A. 1995b. A model for circadian oscillations in the *Drosophila* period protein (PER). *Proceedings of the Royal Society of London. B: Biological Sciences* 261 (1362):319–324.

Golden, S., M. Ishiura, C.H. Johnson, and T. Kondo. 1997. Cyanobacterial circadian rhythms. *Annual Review of Plant Physiology and Plant Molecular Biology* 48:327–354.

Grush, R. 2004. The emulation theory of representation: Motor control, imagery, and perception. *Behavioral and Brain Sciences* 27:377–396.

Hagler, D.J. and M.I. Sereno. 2006. Spatial maps in frontal and prefrontal cortex. *NeuroImage* 29:567–577.

Hannibal, J., P. Hindersson, S.M. Knudsen, B. Georg, and J. Fahrenkrug. 2002. The photopigment melanopsin is exclusively present in pituitary adenylate cyclase-activating polypeptide-containing retinal ganglion cells of the retinohypothalamic tract. *Journal of Neuroscience* 22:1–7.

Hardin, P.E., J.C. Hall, and M. Rosbash. 1990. Feedback of the *Drosophila period* gene product on circadian cycling of its messenger rna levels. *Nature* 343 (6258):536–540.

Haselager, P., A. de Groot, and H. van Rappard. 2003. Representationalism vs. anti-representationalism: a debate for the sake of appearance. *Philosophical Psychology* 16:5–23.

Hatori, M., H. Le, C. Vollmers, S.R. Keding, N. Tanaka, C. Schmedt, T. Jegla, and S. Pand. 2008. Inducible ablation of melanopsin-expressing retinal ganglion cells reveals their central role in non-image forming visual responses. *PLoS ONE* 3 (6):e2451.

Hattar, S., R.J. Lucas, N. Mrosovsky, S. Thompson, R.H. Douglas, M.W. Hankins, J. Lem, M. Biel, F. Hofmann, R.G. Foster, and K.-W. Yau. 2003. Melanopsin and rod-cone photoreceptive systems account for all major accessory visual functions in mice. *Nature* 424 (6944):75–81.

Henschen, S.E. 1893. On the visual path and centre. *Brain* 16:170–180.

Herzog, E.D., S.J. Aton, R. Numano, Y. Sakaki, and H. Tei. 2004. Temporal precision in the mammalian circadian system: A reliable clock from less reliable neurons. *Journal of Biological Rhythms* 19 (1):35–46.

Holmes, G.M. 1918. Disturbances of visual orientation. *British Journal of Ophthalmology* 2:449–468.

Honma, S. and K.-I. Honma. 1999. Light-induced uncoupling of multioscillatory circadian system in a diurnal rodent, asian chipmunk. *American Journal of Physiology: Regulatory, Integrative, and Comparative Physiology* 276 (5):R1390–1396.

Hubel, D.H. and T.N. Wiesel. 1962. Receptive fields, binocular interaction and functional architecture in the cat's visual cortex. *Journal of Physiology* 160:106–154.

Hubel, D.H. and T.N. Wiesel. 1968. Receptive fields and functional architecture of monkey striate cortex. *Journal of Physiology* 195:215–243.

Inouye, T. 1909. *Die Sehstörungen bei Schussverletzungen der kortikalen Sehsphäre nach Beobachtungen an Verwundeten der letzten japanischen Kriege*. Engelmann.

Jackson, J.H. 1884. Evolution and dissolution of the nervous system. *Lancet* 123:555–558, 649–652, 739–744.

Kalsbeek, A., I.F. Palm, S.E. La Fleur, F.A.J.L. Scheer, S. Perreau-Lenz, M. Ruiter, F. Kreier, C. Cailotto, and R.M. Buijes. 2006. SCN outputs and the hypothalamic balance of life. *Journal of Biological Rhythms* 21 (6):458–469.

King, D.P., Y. Zhao, A.M. Sangoram, L.D. Wilsbacher, M. Tanaka, M.P. Antoch, T.D. Steeves, M.H. Vitaterna, J.M. Kornhauser, P.L. Lowrey, F.W. Turek, and J.S. Takahashi. 1997. Positional cloning of the mouse circadian *Clock* gene. *Cell* 89 (4):641–653.

Konopka, R.J. and S. Benzer. 1971. Clock mutants of *Drosophila melanogaster*. *Proceedings of the National Academy of Sciences (USA)* 89:2112–2116.

Kramer, A., F.-C. Yang, P. Snodgrass, X. Li, T.E. Scammell, F.C Davis, and C.J. Weitz. 2001. Regulation of daily locomotor activity and sleep by hypothalamic EGF receptor signaling. *Science* 294 (5551):2511–2515.

Kuffler, S. W. 1953. Discharge patterns and functional organization of mammalian retina. *Journal of Neurophysiology* 16:37–68.

Lehman, M.N., R. Silver, W.R. Gladstone, R.M. Kahn, M. Gibson, and E.L. Bittman. 1987. Circadian rhythmicity restored by neural transplant. Immunocytochemical characterization of the graft and its integration with the host brain. *Journal of Neuroscience* 7 (6):1626–1638.

Leyton, A.S.F. and C.S. Sherrington. 1917. Observations on the excitable cortex of the chimpanzee, orang-utan and gorilla. *Quarterly Journal of Experimental Physiology* 11:135–222.

Merzenich, M.M. and J.F. Brugge. 1973. Representation of the cochlear partition on the superior temporal plane of the macaque monkey. *Brain Research* 50:275–296.

Millikan, R.G. 1984. *Language, thought, and other biological categories*. MIT Press.

Mitsui, S., S. Yamaguchi, T. Matsuo, Y. Ishida, and H. Okamura. 2001. Antagonistic role of E4BP4 and PAR proteins in the circadian oscillatory mechanism. *Genes & Development* 15 (8):995–1006.

Moore, R.Y. and V.B. Eichler. 1972. Loss of a circadian adrenal corticosterone rhythm following suprachiasmatic lesions in the rat. *Brain Research* 42:201–206.

Munk, H. 1881. *Über die Funktionen der Großhirnrinde*. Hirschwald.

Nakahata, Y., M. Kaluzova, B. Grimaldi, S. Sahar, J. Hirayama, D. Chen, L.P. Guarente, and P. Sassone-Corsi. 2008. The NAD^+-dependent deacetylase SIRT1 modulates CLOCK-mediated chromatin remodeling and circadian control. *Cell* 134 (2):329–340.

Nielsen, K. 2010. Representation and dynamics. *Philosophical Psychology* 23.

Panda, S., M.P. Antoch, B.H. Miller, A.I. Su, A.B. Schook, M. Straume, P.G. Schultz, S.A. Kay, J.S. Takahashi, and J.B. Hogenesch. 2002. Coordinated transcription of key pathways in the mouse by the circadian clock. *Cell* 109 (3):307–320.

Panda, S., I. Provencio, D.C. Tu, S.S. Pires, M.D. Rollag, A.M. Castrucci, M.T. Pletcher, T.K. Sato, T. Wiltshire, M. Andahazy, S. Kay, R.N. van Gelder, and J.B. Hogenesch. 2003. Melanopsin is required for non-image-forming photic responses in blind mice. *Science* 301 (5632):525–527.

Penfield, W. and E. Boldrey. 1937. Somatic motor and sensory representation in the cerebral cortex of man as studied by electrical stimulation. *Brain* 60:389–443.

Pittendrigh, C.S. 1960–1961. On temporal organization in living systems. *Harvey Lectures* 56:93–125.

Plautz, J.D., M. Kaneko, J.C. Hall, and S.A. Kay. 1997. Independent photoreceptive circadian clocks throughout *Drosophila*. *Science* 278 (5343):1632–1635.

Provencio, I., G. Jiang, W.J. De Grip, W.P. Hayes, and M.D. Rollag. 1998. Melanopsin: An opsin in melanophores, brain, and eye. *Proceedings of the National Academy of Sciences* 95 (1):340–345.

Provencio, I., M.D. Rollag, and A.M. Castrucci. 2002. Anatomy: Photoreceptive net in the mammalian retina. *Nature* 415 (6871):493–493.

Pulivarthy, S.R., N. Tanaka, D.K. Welsh, L. De Haro, I.M. Verma, and S. Panda. 2007. Reciprocity between phase shifts and amplitude changes in the mammalian circadian clock. *Proceedings of the National Academy of Sciences* 104 (51):20356–20361.

Ralph, M.R., R.G. Foster, F.C. Davis, and M. Menaker. 1990. Transplanted suprachiasmatic nucleus determines circadian period. *Science* 247 (4945):975–978.

Ruiz-Mirazo, K., J. Peretó, and A. Moreno. 2004. A universal definition of life: Autonomy and open-ended evolution. *Origins of Life and Evolution of the Biosphere* 34:323–346.

Rutter, J., M. Reick, L.C. Wu, and S.L. McKnight. 2001. Regulation of Clock and NPAS2 DNA binding by the redox state of NAD cofactors. *Science* 293 (5529):510–514.

Saper, C.B., G. Cano, and T.E. Scammell. 2005. Homeostatic, circadian, and emotional regulation of sleep. *Journal of Comparative Neurology* 43 (1):92–98.

Sawaki, Y., I. Nihonmatsu, and H. Kawamura. 1984. Transplantation of the neonatal suprachiasmatic nuclei into rats with complete bilateral suprachiasmatic lesions. *Neuroscience Research* 1 (1):67–72.

Schaap, J., H. Albus, H.T. van der Leest, P.H.C. Eilers, L. Détári, and J.H. Meijer. 2003. Heterogeneity of rhythmic suprachiasmatic nucleus neurons: Implications for circadian waveform and photoperiodic encoding. *Proceedings of the National Academy of Sciences of the United States of America* 100 (26):15994–15999.

Sereno, M.I. 2001. Mapping of contralateral space in retinotopic coordinates by a parietal cortical area in humans. *Science* 294:1350–1354.

Shigeyoshi, Y., K. Taguchi, S. Yamamoto, S. Takekida, L. Yan, H. Tei, T. Moriya, S. Shibata, J.J. Loros, J.C. Dunlap, and H. Okamura. 1997. Light-induced resetting of a mammalian circadian clock is associated with rapid induction of the mPer1 transcript. *Cell* 91 (7):1043–1053.

Silver, R., J. LeSauter, P.A. Tresco, and M.N. Lehman. 1996. A diffusible coupling signal from the transplanted suprachiasmatic nucleus controlling circadian locomotor rhythms. *Nature* 382 (6594):810–813.

Siwicki, K.K., C. Eastman, G. Petersen, M. Rosbash, and J.C. Hall. 1988. Antibodies to the period gene product of *Drosophila* reveal diverse tissue distribution and rhythmic changes in the visual system. *Neuron* 1:141–150.

Stephan, F.K., J.M. Swann, and C.L. Sisk. 1979. Entrainment of circadian rhythms by feeding schedules in rats with suprachiasmatic lesions. *Behavioral and Neural Biology* 25 (4):545–554.

Stephan, F.K. and I. Zucker. 1972. Circadian rhythms in drinking behavior and locomotor activity of rats are eliminated by hypothalamic lesions. *Proceedings of the National Academy of Sciences (USA)* 69:1583–1586.

Storch, K.-F., O. Lipan, I. Leykin, N. Viswanathan, F.C. Davis, W.H. Wong, and C.J. Weitz. 2002. Extensive and divergent circadian gene expression in liver and heart. *Nature* 417 (6884):78–83.

Strogatz, S.H. 2001. Exploring complex networks. *Nature* 410 (6825):268–276.

Sun, Z.S., U. Albrecht, O. Zhuchenko, J. Bailey, G. Eichele, and C.C. Lee. 1997. RIGUI, a putative mammalian ortholog of the *Drosophila period* gene. *Cell* 90 (6):1003–1011.

Talbot, S.A. and W.H. Marshall. 1941. Physiological studies on neural mechanisms of visual localization and discrimination. *American Journal of Ophthalmology* 24:1255–1263.

Travnickova-Bendova, Z., N. Cermakian, S.M. Reppert, and P. Sassone-Corsi. 2002. Bimodal regulation of mPeriod promoters by CREB-dependent signaling and CLOCK/BMAL1 activity. *Proceedings of the National Academy of Sciences of the United States of America* 99 (11):7728–7733.

van der Leest, H.T., T. Houben, S. Michel, T. Deboer, H. Albus, M.J. Vansteensel, G.D. Block, and J.H. Meijer. 2007. Seasonal encoding by the circadian pacemaker of the SCN. *Current Biology* 17 (5):468–473.

van Gelder, T. 1995. What might cognition be, if not computation? *Journal of Philosophy* 92:345–381.

van Leeuwen, C. 2007. Small world networks and the brain. *The Brain and Neural Networks* 14 (3):186–197.

Vitaterna, M.H., D.P. King, A.-M. Chang, J.M. Kornhauser, P.L. Lowrey, J.D. McDonald, W.F. Dove, L.H. Pinto, F.W. Turek, and J.S. Takahashi. 1994. Mutagenesis and mapping of a mouse gene, *Clock*, essential for circadian behavior. *Science* 264 (5159):719–725.

Welsh, D.K., D.E. Logothetis, M. Meister, and S.M. Reppert. 1995. Individual neurons dissociated from rat suprachiasmatic nucleus express independently phased circadian firing rhythms. *Neuron* 14 (4):697–706.

Welsh, D.K., J.S. Takahashi, and S.A. Kay. 2010. Suprachiasmatic nucleus: Cell autonomy and network properties. *Annual Review of Physiology* 72 (1).

Wernicke, C. 1874. *Der aphasische Symptomenkomplex: Eine psychologische Studie auf anatomischer Basis*. Cohn and Weigert.

Winfree, A.T. 1970. Integrated view of resetting a circadian clock. *Journal of Theoretical Biology* 28 (3):327–374.

Woolsey, C.N. 1943. "Second" somatic receiving areas in the cerebral cortex of cat, dog, and monkey. *Federation Proceedings* 2:55.

Woolsey, C.N. and E.M. Walzl. 1942. Topical projection of nerve fibers from local regions of the cochlea to the cerebral cortex of the cat. *Bulletin of the Johns Hopkins Hospital* 71:315–344.

Yamazaki, S., R. Numano, M. Abe, A. Hida, R. Takahashi, M. Ueda, G.D. Block, Y. Sakaki, M. Menaker, and H. Tei. 2000. Resetting central and peripheral circadian oscillators in transgenic rats. *Science* 288 (5466):682–685.

Yoo, S.-H., S. Yamazaki, P.L. Lowrey, K. Shimomura, C.H. Ko, E.D. Buhr, S.M. Siepka, H.K. Hong, W.J. Oh, O.J. Yoo, M. Menaker, and J.S. Takahashi. 2004. PERIOD2::LUCIFERASE real-time reporting of circadian dynamics reveals persistent circadian oscillations in mouse peripheral tissues. *Proceedings of the National Academy of Sciences* 101 (15):5339–5346.

Zylka, M.J., L.P. Shearman, D.R. Weaver, and S.M. Reppert. 1998. Three *period* homologs in mammals: Differential light responses in the suprachiasmatic circadian clock and oscillating transcripts outside of brain. *Neuron* 20 (6):1103–1110.

8

The Explanatory Value of Representations in Cognitive Neuroscience

KAI VOGELEY & ANDREAS BARTELS

8.1 Introduction

The paper tries to elucidate the role of the concept of representation in cognitive neuroscientific explanations. Are representations necessary to explain mental phenomena, or is it possible to replace them without loss by representation-free explanations as proposed by the dynamic systems approach?[1] In order to answer this question, it will be necessary to clarify (Section 8.2) how cognitive neuroscientific explanations can be classified with respect to the recent debate about the concept of explanation in the philosophy of science. Do neuroscientific explanations constitute *mechanistic explanations* of some kind (Machamer et al. 2000, Bechtel 2008) or rather some sort of *inferential explanations* (either in form of the traditional covering law model or in form of Woodward's (2000) model of causal explanation based on invariant generalization)? If they are mechanistic explanations of some kind, *how* do

---

[1]It should be mentioned that dynamical systems approaches are not *per se* committed to representation-free explanations. It is completely possible to combine non-representational explanations referring to fundamental dynamical equations governing an idealized model of an actual complex neural system, with some representational interpretation referring to higher-level structures that emerge from that fundamental dynamics (Colin Allen by personal communication; cf. also Bechtel 2001a).

Knowledge and Representation.
Albert Newen, Andreas Bartels
& Eva-Maria Jung (eds.).
Copyright © 2011, CSLI Publications.

mechanisms explain? We will argue that cognitive neuroscientific explanations can be understood as mechanistic explanations which explain by presenting and connecting causal patterns—and are thus compatible with Woodward's model of causal explanation.

Section 8.3 asks what concept of representation fits best with the requirements of cognitive neuroscientific research and argues in favor of a functional role concept of representation (Bartels and May 2009). In order to test and scrutinize these theses further, in Section 8.4 we shall discuss recent studies in social cognitive neuroscience from our own group (Kuzmanovic et al. 2009). The case of gaze behavior as an important signaling system in social cognition demonstrates, firstly, that representational content should, in general, be understood as determined by the functional role of the representation (as opposed to the causal-correlative account) and, secondly, that the use of representational assumptions allows investigators to explain how subjects can extract and react to relevant information from the environment, in our case information about other persons and the relationship between oneself and the other person. Finally (Section 8.5), we analyze how, in general, representations—understood as functional roles—do explanatory work in cognitive neuroscience. The result is that representational explanations are a special type of mechanistic explanations, characterized by information processing mechanisms. What makes them distinct is their particular explanatory interest: to show how information about the outer world enables a subject to successfully navigate through the physical and social world.

8.2   How do Mechanisms in Cognitive Neuroscience Explain?

The recent debate on explanation focuses on the question: which *type* of explanation characterizes the explanatory practices in the special sciences such as cognitive neuroscience? Several philosophers emphazise the stark contrast between *nomological* and *mechanistic* explanations. Bechtel, for instance, claims that

> [...] instead of abstracting general principles and applying them to specific cases, researchers focus from the beginning on the specifics of the composition and organization of a mechanism that generates a particular form of behavior. (Bechtel 2008, 4)

The main reason the proponents of mechanistic explanation put forward for abandoning nomological (or: covering law) explanation is that in the special sciences there are simply no laws available to explain particular phenomena of interest. To be sure, there are laws (e.g., chemical and physical laws) that provide the background against which, in the case of neuroscience, brain processes develop their characteristic activities or operations. But it is not these enabling background laws that serve to explain specifically cognitive or mental phenomena. Rather these laws specify regularities in some of the operations within mechanisms by showing how specific variables are related mathematically. The explanatory focus lies on the concrete operations or activities that produce the cognitive or mental phenomenon. Special sciences like cognitive neuroscience do not involve, critics of nomological explanation claim, special laws but only specific arrangements of entities and activities which may in turn be characterized in terms of laws of more basic level sciences.

But how does the focus on the 'specifics of the composition and organization' of a mechanism produce explanations in the special sciences? If there are no specific laws to do the explanatory work, what else takes their place? To be sure, just specifying which entities, relations, and operations constitute a mechanism will not be sufficient in order to show how the mechanism explains a certain phenomenon. There are, roughly, two opposing views concerning the explanatory value of mechanisms. The first view, taken among others by Bechtel, we will call the 'functionalist' view of mechanistic explanation; the second view proposed by, for instance, Machamer and Craver we call the 'production' view. According to the functionalist view "a mechanism is a structure performing a function in virtue of its component parts, component operations, and their organization" (Bechtel 2008, 13). Nature does not reveal such structures by itself, rather a particular structure is discovered through what Bechtel calls 'structural decomposition' (decomposition of the mechanism into its parts) and 'functional decomposition' (decomposition into operations) (Bechtel 2008, 14). The relevant components and operations characterizing a mechanism have to be identified by means of a functional analysis (cf. Cummins 1975) with respect to their contributions to the final production of the phenomenon to be explained.

To explain a phenomenon by the workings of a mechanism involves the specification of a series of *causal relations* connecting the changes occurring at, or with, some components of the mechanism and, finally, the statement of a *constitution* (or realization) relation between the final result of the mechanism at the micro-level of its causal operations (e.g., neural processes) and the macro-phenomenon to be explained (e.g., mental or cognitive phenomenon). For instance, a mechanistic explanation of how you are able to listen to a lecture and take notes proceeds by saying that hearing the lecture caused chemical changes in your brain, as a result of electrical signals that are transmitted through your hippocampus, the effect on the hippocampus consisting in changes in the concentrations of various chemicals at the synapses between cells, etc., until we reach a brain condition that constitutes remembering the content of the lecture (cf. Bechtel 2008, 154).

In contrast, according to the 'production' view (e.g., Machamer et al. 2000, Craver 2008), mechanistic explanations differ from inferential explanations (explanations by means of laws or invariant generalizations) by their particular autonomous explanatory role of the operations or 'activities' of a mechanism. Machamer, for instance, claims that "activities are the producers of change", whereas "entities are the things that engage in activities" (Machamer et al. 2000, 3). Now, those activities, for instance the activity of the neurotransmitter and receptor binding, are based on properties of the entities engaged, in that case, the structural properties and charge distributions of the neurotransmitter and its receptor (cf. Machamer et al. 2000, 3). But mechanistic explanations do not rely on these basic properties and laws formulating relations between them, but on the more specific activities themselves. Since there are no laws that formulate how these specific activities operate, the activities rather replace the laws in their explanatory role. But how can activities explain by themselves? How can "mechanisms do things", as Machamer et al. (2000) claim? This seems to presuppose the existence of some intrinsic productivity or 'productive nature' of an activity, such that the activities which are present in a mechanism, spontaneously unfold their specific productivity producing the results of the mechanism.

Can we understand this notion of mechanistic explanation in a way that does not commit us to that metaphysics of activities? We think yes. Take the *activities* constituting a mechanism as *functional roles* performed by the entities of a mechanism. This conforms to what Machamer et al. say about activities: "Functions are the roles played by entities and activities in the mechanism ... [T]o see an activity as a function is to see it as a component in some mechanism" (Machamer et al. 2000, 6). If activities are to be conceived of as functions and functions are just roles played by activities within a mechanism, then this means that activities can be individuated by their (functional) roles within a mechanism. For instance, the phenomenon of binding of neurotransmitter molecules to a specific receptor plays a functional role as a component of the mechanism of chemical neurotransmission, and it is exactly this role that characterizes the respective activity as a component of the mechanism. In other words, processes occurring in a mechanism are particular activities playing a definite role in that mechanism.

From that perspective, the necessary connection between an activity and its productivity (how the activity works within the mechanism) no longer needs to involve a strong metaphysical assumption, but simply follows from the fact that functional role characterizations of an entity by their very nature pick out that entity with respect to its functional contribution within a mechanism (cf. Mumford 2003)—in our case, with respect to its productivity.

In light of a functional role reading of 'activities' the distinction between the 'functionalist' and the 'production' view of mechanistic explanation reduces to a terminological matter. Explanation by means of productive activities, according to this reading, has to be taken as explanation by means of processes characterized by their functional role within a mechanism. Even the seemingly incompatible view proposed by Machamer et al. according to which providing a description of a mechanism for a phenomenon *is* to explain that phenomenon, can be made compatible with the functionalist view. By a 'description of a mechanism' Machamer means a representation of a series of sub-processes (or activities), where each process in the series includes changes in entities of the mechanism that are causally related to each other. As we already mentioned with respect to Bechtel's conception of mechanistic explanation, the changes occurring in a mechanism are connected by causal relations. In a 'description' of a mechanism, therefore, causal relations have to be necessarily included.

In sum, we propose the following thesis: a mechanism is composed of sub-processes (that can either be described as 'activities' or as 'functional roles') which include changes in entities connected by causal relations. The sub-processes themselves are connected by causal relations—those causal relations that lead from the change that occurs at the end of one sub-process to the change occurring at the beginning of another sub-process.[2] It turns out that the causal description and the functional role description of a mechanism are complementary formats of description working on different levels of description: whereas causal notions govern the fundamental, relatively fine-grained level, functional role terminology works on a higher, more coarse-grained level.

Since causal relations, as they occur in neural mechanisms, are specific relations that depend on the mechanism concerned, they will, in general, not be represented by fundamental laws but by invariant generalizations (cf. Woodward 2000). Woodward's model of causal explanation is explicitly directed at the requirements and constraints for

---

[2]Note that what we describe here are local connections between single sub-processes. Nothing is implied by this about the global structure built by the totality of sub-processes. In particular, we do not presuppose a linear structure.

mechanistic explanations in the special sciences, so it is much better suited than the traditional nomological approach to explicate how causal relations are modeled within mechanisms. Causal explanation, Woodward claims, has nothing to do with subsumption under (causal) laws, but rather

> [...] with the exhibition of patterns of counterfactual dependence of a special sort, involving *active* counterfactuals—counterfactuals the antecedents of which are made true by interventions. Only invariant generalizations will support active counterfactuals—hence the connection between explanation and invariance. (Woodward 2000, 199)

Thus, the Woodward approach to causal explanation contains, firstly, the claim that to explain is to refer to causes (or to state causal relations), secondly, the claim that a cause appears in the model as an intervention on some variable X which is counterfactually connected to a corresponding change in some other variable Y (which change represents what we call the 'effect' of the 'cause'), and, thirdly, the claim that causal statements referring to a counterfactual relation between X and Y must be based on invariant generalizations (represented by recursive equations including the variables X and Y), i.e., the general relation between variables X and Y must be stable with respect to interventions in a definite range of numerical values and also with respect to a definite range of changes in the external conditions (cf. Woodward 2000, 205f.).

To summarize, a statement of a mechanism in cognitive neuroscience as well as in other 'special sciences' explains by exhibiting causal patterns, i.e., patterns of counterfactual dependence which are not based on laws of nature, but only on stable, invariant generalizations.[3] Those causal patterns make up the core of the causal sub-processes that constitute the mechanism. The mechanistic explanation is completed by connecting the single sub-processes (activities) either to a series that leads from the initial conditions to some termination conditions or to a net of components with some complex, non-linear dynamics.

8.3 Which Concept of Representation for Cognitive Neuroscience?

In cognitive neuroscience, the concept of representation is predominantly used in its *causal-correlative* sense. It is widely assumed that the preference for this concept of representation is not accidental, but reflects the methodological needs of neuroscientific research. We shall

---

[3]Those generalizations may be very weak in some cases, i.e., the generalization may merely extend over a small range of parameter values.

argue that this assessment tells only one half of the truth. The full truth is that neuroscientific explanations favor a functional role concept of representation that can be substituted only in a fraction of cases by its 'first approximation', the causal-correlative concept of representation. States or processes of a neural system S are representational, according to the causal-correlative reading, if they (a) include causal information about the external states, processes or events that have caused them, and (b) this causal information is used by S as a means of behavioral control. Representations are thus characterized by two aspects: first, they are "information-bearing states" (Bechtel 2001b, 336), and second, the system S in which they occur is 'designed' (in case of organisms by their evolutionary history) to use the information which they are endowed with to direct its exchange with the environment. This aspect has been prominently emphazised by Ruth G. Millikan and Bechtel:

> In its most basic sense, a representation is something (an event or process) that stands in for and carries information about what it represents, enabling the system in which it occurs to use that information in directing its behavior. (Bechtel 2001b, 334)

According to the causal-correlative account, the informational (or representational) content of a particular representational state is characterized by the external state, process or event that has caused it. It is this external state, process or event the representational state bears information about.

A famous philosophical account of how correlations between environmental and internal events endow events of neural activity with informational content has been proposed by Fred Dretske (1981, 1988a). The key idea is that there is a spectrum of possible states $s_1, \ldots, s_n$ of some brain entity that corresponds to a spectrum of external states $e_1, \ldots, e_n$ such that the occurrence of brain state s_i is caused by, and thereby carries information about, the presence of external state e_i. Dretske's account seems to fit exactly with part of the methodological practice of a cognitive neuroscientist studying the information processing by the human brain: the neuroscientist in a first step of his analysis of a mental phenomenon has to search for correlations between neural patterns of activity and events in the external world because these correlations provide the informational content of neural receptor units at the brain–world interface. Bechtel claims that this methodological orientation is a particular characteristic that distinguishes neuroscience from cognitive science:

Cognitive science accounts begin by positing vehicles that figure in information processing operations and then attempt to relate these causally to their contents. In contrast, neuroscientists identify vehicles as a result of the causal processes linking neural processes to sensory and motor systems. Their causal link to content is therefore already secured. (Bechtel 2008, 178)

[The] neuroscientific strategy for identifying representations in the brain is relatively straightforward. Researchers seek to determine what sensory stimulus or motor response is causally linked with the activity of particular neurons. (Bechtel 2008, 186)

If some cell or neural complex is exclusively responding to a certain, e.g., auditory stimulus, then the meaning or informational content it is endowed with by means of this correlation is specified to be *information about the presence of this, e.g., auditory, signal.* Until these basic informational contents of receptor units have been determined, researchers normally do not take the further step of analyzing the connections to other neural subsystems that are engaged in subsequent steps of processing this particular, e.g., auditory, information.

Although the causal-correlative account of representation fits the very first and superficial methodological needs for the analysis of information processing in the brain, it turns out not to be useful for the analysis of informational content at deeper levels of brain activity for the following reasons.[4] First, the individual neurons do not 'know' to what sort of signal they respond. That means, the 'stuff' of the information processed in the brain (electrical and chemical signals), does not bear in itself any mark that could distinguish, for instance, auditory from visual information. Thus, the distinction has to be made by the functional organization—the input and output units, and the connections between the different regions of the brain involved in a particular mode of information processing. The analysis of the informational content of a certain brain unit, therefore, must be a comprehensive functional analysis (cf. Cummins 1975) from an "information processing perspective" (Bechtel 2008, 17). From this perspective the external "target" (e.g., the auditory signal that is processed) refers to only one component of the whole to be analyzed. The particular contribution of neural activity to the emergence of a mental phenomenon as a whole, i.e., the functional role of the neural process with respect to the production of

---

[4]We are talking about different "levels" of brain activity here for the sake of simplification. We do not want to imply that we are arguing in favor of a simple linear input-output model of the brain. In fact, recent insights into the robust intrinsic connectivity of the human brain (Raichle et al. 2001) support the view that the brain is driven by a high degree of endogeneous or intrinsic activity.

the mental or cognitive phenomenon, makes up its informational (representational) content[5]—and this sort of content cannot be expressed simply in terms of causal connections to the outer informational source. Brain lesion studies conducted in clinical neuropsychology demonstrate that brain processes can often be understood as modular such that if one process is incomplete or drops out entirely, a particular aspect of the whole mental phenomenon is missing, while other aspects are preserved. In those cases we are tempted to identify the content, i.e., the functional role, of a brain unit by identifying that missing aspect.[6]

In particular, representational contents at different levels of brain activity are specific—determined by the particular task that is accomplished by the components involved at that level. Thus, the contents of receptor subsystems at the early levels or during early steps of processing—even if they can be reconstructed according to the causal-correlative concept of representational content—will not be significant for the deeper levels of processing; they would not be 'carried through' all these levels. To put it in other terms: there are no brain symbols with permanent meanings that would provide a sort of basic vocabulary for the processing activity of the brain at its various levels. The brain, in other words, is not "semantically transparent"(cf. Clark 1989).[7]

Second, causal-correlative accounts are often accused of not being able to cope with the problem of misrepresentation. For their philosophical proponents this was reason enough to supplement their approaches by some sort of teleofunctional or normal condition component. Even if practicing neuroscientists do not notice this problem, when they proceed to talk about representations in the causal-correlative sense, this does not cause any significant damage to their research. The problem of

---

[5]By "neural activity" we are not referring to a rigid concept of brain processes in a given brain region that could be studied in isolation, but to a dynamic concept of neural networks that can be explored and studied in different subsets. How the "relevant" neural networks are to be individuated crucially depends on the functional role under study.

[6]Neuroscientifically, it is important not to neglect the phenomenon of neuroplasticity as variability over time due to impressive adaptive capacities of the brain, even in adulthood. Patients suffering from neurological and/or neuropsychological symptoms on the basis of lesioned brains can recover to often enough impressive degrees, but this has clear limits. The issue of plasticity does not affect the principal line of argumentation presented here.

[7]The way brains code information presumably is not at all related to any sort of processing symbols in the sense that the brain activity itself would allow inferences about the representational contents. In contrast, we are inclined to assume that in each individual brain information is coded in a highly individualized way that is probably best described by connectionist models and dynamic systems theory. However, the way we characterize representation does not contradict the option of a connectionist implementation in the brain.

misrepresentation is simply of no great methodological significance, as long as early levels of information processing are concerned. For neural receptor subsystems indicating the presence or absence of a specified outer signal the problem of misrepresentation reduces to the problem of specifying correctness conditions for the contents of receptor subsystem activities, i.e., of specifying 'intended' targets. As soon as the neuroscientist finds out some 'normal conditions' under which those activities are present, misrepresentation can be explicated as the firing of the receptor caused by 'inadequate' targets, in other words, conditions that are not normal, but still evoke the firing pattern. Another type of misrepresentation would relate to the failure of firing although the 'adequate target' is present and conditions are normal. Thereby the scientist, consciously or not, anticipates a common philosophical solution to the problem.

With increasing complexity of information processing in the brain, misrepresentation becomes a richer and methodologically more interesting phenomenon. What is represented by a certain brain activity can no longer be discovered by singling out some 'preferred' sort of objects causing the representation under normal conditions, but will be, in general, a certain aspect of a comprehensive mental phenomenon. Thus, the analysis of 'correct' and 'incorrect' representations will be unsuccessful if only different possible causes for the presence of the brain activity are examined. Only a detailed functional analysis of a greater complex of representations to which the particular representation belongs as a component can elucidate the phenomenon of a misrepresentation. This analysis often proceeds by studying deficits of brain functions. Cases of misrepresentation provide the best evidence for the need to include the functional role into the conceptualization of brain activities, the mere fact that misrepresentations can occur shows that a functional role concept of representation is necessary and the only adequate way to properly understand and explain brain function. The notion of misrepresentation then gets a functional meaning: the particular brain activity does not perform its normal functional role, the normal role being uncovered by the dropout of the activity within an organized mechanism. Thus, we see that there is a concrete need to use a functional role concept of informational (representational) content—a concept that allows a neat specification of misrepresentation—if complex sorts of brain processing are the subject of research. If we understand "functional role" in the sense of Cummins' functional analysis, content explanations in which content is conceived of as functional role, are not threatened by trivialization. The contribution of a functional component of a system does in a non-trivial way (partly) explain a certain resulting capacity of the system. Misrepresentation can be conceptualized, according to functional analysis, as the non-occurrence or malfunction of a component of the system, with the result that the 'normal' resulting capacity of the system does not occur. This conceptualization presupposes that the functional analysis addresses some normal capacity of a system. Since the task of cognitive neuroscientific research typically consists in the analysis of a particular cognitive or social capacity of a system, this in no way undermines the concept of misrepresentation as conceived in functional analysis. The only problem that could arise would be that the contribution of some functional role would be 'too near' to the capacity of the system to be explained. What follows then, is an almost or completely trivial explanation, but this sort of accident threatens all sorts of explanations, not only representational and functional role explanations in particular (see Bartels and May 2009, 72f.).

To summarize, contrary to the first impression, the methodological problems of neuroscientific research cannot be successfully tackled with a causal-correlative concept of representation. The informational content realized by brain processes can only be discovered by means of proper functional analyses of the system to which those processes belong. Misrepresentation plays a key-role in this analysis: conjectures about the function of a certain component of the system can only be tested by means of the consequences following a dropout of this component.[8] The component then does not work in the way it works within the ideally correct working system; it does not provide its normal representational contribution to the mental phenomena produced by the cognitive system. From the case of misrepresentation we can learn what the normal contribution of the unit is. This is the understanding of misrepresentation that has to be presupposed in order to test functional assumptions as needed in the functional analysis-methodology in cognitive neuroscience. The functional role concept of representation constitutes the background for the explication of this notion of misrepresentation, and by applying this notion, the functional analysis of representational contents can be actually carried out.

---

[8]By stating this, we do not want to defend a simple "modular" concept that would imply that a lesion of a brain region would always and in every case lead to a characteristic "standard" cognitive or functional deficit. In contrast, we have to assume that the relation between the nervous system as a whole and its sub-components is complex, presumably because of the integrated design of the nervous system and because of the high degree of individualized wiring patterns that are the result of a complex interaction between the genetic disposition and environmental imprinting processes that are reflected in the brain architecture.

Examples of simple feedback systems like the Watt governor, exploited by Bechtel (2001b, 2008), that exemplify the causal-correlative notion of representation are in a sense misleading, if taken as representative for representation in the neurosciences in general. It presents, as mentioned before, only half of the truth:

> [W]hen techniques such as single-cell recording and neuroimaging are employed to understand how the brain performs cognitive tasks, implicitly the notion of representation on which they are relying is the same as I invoked in identifying representations in the Watt governor. (Bechtel 2001b, 334)

The true part of this statement is that the Watt governor shows how the components of a system (in that case: the spindle arms) can carry information about other parts of the system (the speed of the flywheel), even if all these components are situated in a closed causal circuit and the workings of them could be described exclusively in physical terms. This shows that (i) representations can be parts of the dynamics of the system (they are not distinct static entities that are somehow separated from the dynamics of the system), and (ii) representational notions apply to the informational aspect of the system that can perfectly coexist with its purely physical aspects. That a system can be described in purely physical terms does not mean that there could not be, in addition to that, some real informational aspect of the working of the system.

The false component in the above statement is that all brain activities can be allegedly subsumed under the notion of detector functions, and thus be correctly understood by the causal-correlative concept of representation. Detectors play their part in the brain, but not all of the representational activity of the brain is a sort of detection. Thus the informational content of a type of representational state cannot, in general, be specified by means of the (normal) cause of that type of state. Contents by causal correlations are only one special case (for Bechtel's concept of representations see Bechtel 2001b, 336). The most general concept of representation for cognitive neuroscience is the functional role concept.[9]

---

[9]We emphasize that both, the causal-correlative and the functional role concept of representation involve a consumer aspect of representation: representational content is essentially *used* by a system (cf. Section 8.3). The difference between the two accounts concerns the way in which representational content is specified.

8.4 Social Neuroscience as a Case for Functional Role Explanation

That causal correlations do not exhaust the notion of representational content can be demonstrated by the results of two recent studies from our own group in the research field of *social (cognitive) neuroscience*. This field can be understood as a subfield of cognitive neuroscience that deals with processes either related to self–other-differentiation or self–other-exchange for the purpose of interaction and/or communication with others (Vogeley and Roepstorff 2009). In the past, these cognitive processes have been dealt with extensively by social psychology. Empirical studies during the last decade focused on these aforementioned processes of self–other-differentiation, often operationalised as self-referential cognition, for instance in spatial cognition (e.g., Vogeley et al. 2004) or with respect to the experience of agency (David et al. 2006, 2008) and self–other-exchange, empirically indicated by classical theory of mind or mentalizing studies (e.g., Vogeley et al. 2001). Converging evidence was provided that—employing functional magnetic resonance imaging (fMRI)—one particular brain region is recruited during the majority of social cognition tasks being studied, namely the so-called medial prefrontal cortex (MPFC) (Amodio and Frith 2006).

A particularly interesting research field is human gaze behavior. Gaze and 'eye-contact' are crucial elements of social interactions. Gaze helps to regulate dyadic encounters, and its coordination can help to establish three-way relations between self, other and the object world. An interesting recent study focusing on person perception was able to distinguish two different subprocesses in the evaluation of social gaze, namely gaze detection and gaze evaluation (Kuzmanovic et al. 2009) by the systematic variation of the experience of being gazed at by virtual characters with different durations. 'Gaze detection', the mere perception of being gazed at, irrespective of the duration with which a virtual character gazed at the participant, is represented by the increased neural activity in the fusiform and temporoparietal cortices (as measured by fMRI), in other words, the functional role of these brain regions is gaze detection in the framework of this particular experimental operationalization. These brain regions are assumed to be responsible for biological motion detection, in this case detection of social gaze. To evaluate the social gaze of the virtual character, subjects had to make a sympathy rating of the virtual character at different durations of directed gaze. Subjects were instructed before the experiment that they would be asked to provide a likeability rating after each trial. In order not to confound brain activities related to motor processes with brain activity related to cognitive processes, the ratings had to be performed directly after perceiving the short animated video sequences. An increase of gaze duration varying between 1 s and 4 s resulted in an increase of the sympathy rating towards the virtual character. This experience was associated with increased neural activity in the MPFC, and we interpreted this phenomenon as 'gaze evaluation'. As the detection of social gaze is a necessary requirement for the successful and adequate interpretation of someone's gaze behavior, gaze detection can be interpreted as an early stage or 'level' of information processing related to social gaze that is essentially based upon information from the sensory input being subsequently processed in the unimodal association cortex of the visual system. In contrast, gaze evaluation can be understood as a late stage or 'level' of processing realized by increased neural activity in the MPFC that has often been found as a neural correlate of social cognitive tasks of this kind (e.g., Amodio and Frith 2006).

Why is gaze evaluation, as opposed to gaze detection, an example of neural vehicles (neural correlates) bearing content that is determined by the functional role played by the correlates? We want to argue that in gaze evaluation, generally speaking, *social information* is extracted from the sensory signals expressed by the virtual character (or a real person involved in a dyadic interaction between two personal agents). The experience or perception of being gazed at is responsible for a certain impression formation or person perception with a particular sort of social evaluation (e.g., sympathy, likeability). What the behavioral data show is that increased duration leads to higher sympathy ratings as compared to shorter durations. This experience is, on the other hand, associated with increased neural activity, essentially in the MPFC. We conclude that the content of this sort of neural activity in the MPFC is exactly this social evaluation attached to person perception for which the neural activity is responsible according to its functional role. In that sense, the MPFC represents gaze evaluation in the framework of this given operationalization. What gives gaze duration its social significance is not any intrinsic social dimension of the informational input, but the fact that the neural correlates located in the MPFC reacting to gaze duration show increased activity that in turn correlates with increased likeability evaluations towards the virtual characters. One might be tempted to say that the increased neural activity caused increased likeability ratings—based on invariant generalizations that can be inferred from empirical observations in this experiment. Thus, the vehicles of the gaze duration representation play their role in causing a certain form of social behavior, depending on the gaze duration signal—and thereby get their definite social meaning. In other words, the social information processed by these correlates is not some sort of intrinsic information somehow joined to the informational source, but is constituted by the social nature of the functional roles played by the neural correlates processing the information.[10] For a person who does not have the capacity to react in that way (for whom gaze duration would not change the experience of sympathy or likeability, for instance) the signal literally has no social informational content. This would then establish a case of *misrepresentation*—the function of the neural correlates is to 'read out' social information of a special kind, but the reading mechanism does not work in the intended way (as is probably the case in autistic persons). The phenomenon of misrepresentation thus indicates what the functional role content for a certain type of representational vehicle is.

Whereas representational vehicles that read social information out of gaze durations have their content determined by their functional role, *detection* of gaze *direction* seems to be, at least partly, a representational task of biological motion detection. The capacity to detect biological motion is associated with increased neural activity in the posterior parts of the superior temporal sulcus (pSTS) which is known to be involved in processing various formats of biological motion (Kuzmanovic et al. 2009, 1159). Motion detectors are paradigmatic examples of a causal-correlative interpretation of content. What is represented is a feature of something 'out there'. Even processing of gaze direction has some social component: direct gaze is associated with an increased likeability of faces in contrast to averted gaze (Kuzmanovic et al. 2009, 1159). But this effect is independent of gaze duration which underlines the assumption that the social content connected to duration evaluation actually constitutes a distinct type of representation. There is empirical evidence that

> [...] gaze duration as compared to gaze direction represents a more complex source of social information because it requires more sophisticated mentalizing abilities in order to perform an adequate interpretation (Kuzmanovic et al. 2009, 1155).

---

[10]In the framework of social neuroscience two different networks of brain regions have been consistently shown to be associated with social cognitive functions, namely the so-called social neural network (SNN) and the so-called human mirror neuron system (hMNS) (Keyser and Gazzola 2007, Lieberman 2007, Vogeley and Roepstorff 2009). Cognitive neuroscience already provides innovative instruments to study the connectivity between brain regions, both based on structural connectivity and on functional or effective connectivity. This needs to be studied in social neuroscience systematically in the near future.

Thus, whereas 4-year olds are already successful in drawing inferences about others' desires from the simple detection of eye direction, the ability to interpret gaze durations is not developed earlier than at the age of 5 or 6 years (Kuzmanovic et al. 2009, 1155). This study clearly shows empirically that the process of gaze detection and gaze evaluation in the framework of person perception and impression formation are two different processes that can be clearly distinguished on a neural level. We suggest that this empirical finding allows to ascribe characteristically different functional roles or representational contents to these sets of brain regions.

In a related study we investigated the phenomenon of joint attention. The ability and motivation to share attention is a unique aspect of human cognition. By directing or following someone else's gaze it is possible to engage in joint attention and to create a shared experience of the world that is different from perceiving it on our own. Joint attention appears to be a crucial developmental step that is a precursor to the subsequent emergence of more complex social cognitive capacities including mentalizing (the capacity to adequately ascribe mental states to others) and language (Mundy 1993, Gopnik et al. 1994, Charman et al. 2000). Impairments of joint attention have been reported to be associated with autistic spectrum disorders (Dawson et al. 2002). Developing the ability to share attention amounts to realigning one's own intentional relations to the world with those of someone else. It is important to note that it has been suggested that the motivation to engage in such triadic relations with others could be a unique element of human cognition that might promote the active engagement in shared, social realities (Tomasello et al. 2005). This data set supports the suggestion that the activation of the MPFC is a crucial component of the social neural network. The special case of self-initiated joint attention leads to a differential increase in reward-related areas representing the uniquely human motivation to engage in the sharing of experiences.

Recently, for the first time we were able to study the neural correlates of the experience of "true" interaction by engaging participants in a joint attention paradigm (Schilbach et al. 2010). For this purpose, a novel interactive paradigm was developed in which the gaze behavior of participants was recorded by an eye-tracking device and was used to contingently control the gaze of a computer-animated virtual character. Based on a particular instruction, participants, however, were convinced that the depicted virtual character was controlled by a real person outside the scanner and that they themselves would really interact "online" with the virtual character. Experimental systematic variations included tasks to lead or to follow the gaze of the virtual character when fixating one of three objects also shown on the screen. The results showed that following someone else's gaze to engage in joint attention resulted in recruitment of the ventral portions of medial prefrontal cortex (MPFC). The MPFC is also known to be involved in the supramodal coordination of perceptual and cognitive processes. A second interesting result was the activation of the ventral striatum of the participants' reward system as correlate of successfully directing someone else's gaze towards an object. This study shows that the experience of joint attention is systematically associated with increased neural activity in the MPFC. Based on the interventionist account of causation (Woodward 2000) it is justified to suggest that joint attention experience appears to rely upon the recruitment of MPFC as corroborated by lesion studies of the medial prefrontal cortex (Shamay-Tsoory et al. 2004, Frith 2007, Bramham et al. 2009). The additional differential increase of neural activity in reward-related brain areas during self-initiated joint attention experiences might reflect the unique human motivation to engage in the sharing of experiences as mentioned before (Tomasello et al. 2005, Schilbach et al. 2010).

As exemplified by these two studies from our own group, the brain region of the MPFC is held to be responsible for a variety of cognitive processes that can be characterized as "inexact, probabilistic, internally generated" (Mitchell 2009, 249) as common denominator based on the common activations patterns of a variety of cognitive functions. These processes comprise (i) a person's introspective awareness of their own personality traits and idiosyncratic dispositions ("self-concept"); (ii) the self experience or introspective awareness of one's own emotions; (iii) positive or negative evaluations of an object, idea, other person or group; and (iv) the ability to infer the thoughts, feelings and desires of other people ("theory of mind", "mentalizing"). It appears particularly interesting that a number of topics at the core of social psychology appear to constitute a natural group of domains that have a common neural basis as suggested by Mitchell (2009). He summarizes that seemingly different cognitive phenomena (including thinking about oneself, accessing one's attitudes, experiencing emotions, inferring other persons' mental states) are all correlated with increased neural activity in one brain region, the MPFC. This evidence suggests that social cognition is a "natural kind". Mitchell concludes that all these processes can be "distinguished from other kinds of cognitive processing" (Mitchell 2009, 249). This plausible and empirically justified speculation thus clearly shows that the identification of a functional core can stimulate the understanding of its underlying basic neural mechanisms (here: the "fuzzy", probabilistic, internally generated cognition as a core of social cognition that is reflected by the consequent recruitment of the MPFC as observed under the constraints of the fMRI method).

8.5 What Place for Representations in Cognitive Neuroscientific Explanation?

The example of gaze behavior and joint attention has made plausible that (informational) contents of complex neural representations should be explicated in terms of their functional roles. But why should the neuroscientist working on an explanation of mental phenomena like reading out social information "hidden" in the gaze behavior of other persons ascribe representational contents to the neural activities probably relevant for the phenomenon? Do we really need the construct of "content" in order to perform our explanatory aims?

A fact that seems to indicate the relevance of contents in neuroscientific explanation is that in their publications neuroscientists actually speak of specific sorts of information about the environment or about other persons, information that is delivered by various neural mechanisms. This information processing view of the workings of the brain has become very common since the days of Marr's seminal work on vision. But such recourse to terminological practices can hardly count as a good argument for the explanatory relevance of contents.

Let us, for a moment, think about what we are left with if the notion of content had been deleted from our example of gaze evaluation. We would be left with the description of the observable neural activities corresponding to the different experimental conditions and with the verbal evaluations of the likeability of the virtual character by the subjects. Ascribing a specific *content* (namely the social content that the person behind the virtual character that looks at the subject is likeable) to the observed neural activities would establish an explanatory *connection* between the neural activities and the corresponding verbal evaluations: Those neural activities perform the functional role of triggering these verbal evaluations—by means of complex and not yet analysed chains of causal relations.[11] The ascription of content, in a sense, generates a theoretical hypothesis, an anticipation of what a detailed analysis of the causal processes between neural entities and verbal behavior could confirm. Ascribing the theoretical concept "content" to certain neural entities is part of a theoretical assessment of empirical phenomena that enables the neuroscientist to develop and generate

---

[11] Note that this hypothesis is about the assumed functional role of certain neural activities. It is not a hypothesis about the cause of those activities. This is true even if the causal mechanism in which, finally, the relevant functional roles have to be placed has not been discovered at that stage.

hypotheses about those phenomena, in our case hypotheses about behavioural manifestations of the activity of these neural entities to be tested in further experiments in the domain of cognitive neuroscience. Thus, assigning content to neural activities is assigning to them a theoretical property in order to set the interplay between predicting and experimental testing going. This theoretical property should not be a 'virtus dormitiva'-property,[12] that is, content ascription should not exhaust itself in the ascription of a disposition to produce the behavior as it is actually observed. Contents would then really have no explanatory power, and there could be no sense of 'misrepresentation'. In the empirical case study of Section 8.4, the content was of the form "that the person is likeable."[13] This content does normally (within a normal neural environment) manifest itself in appropriate evaluation behavior. But the same content could be present in cases in which a malfunction in behavioral control occurs with the result that the appropriate evaluation behavior fails to appear. The content is not connected to the behavior with analytic necessity. Thus the explanation of the (normal) behavior by means of that content is not true by definition.

For now, it should be clear that informational contents have to be ascribed to relevant neural entities in order to be able to formulate hypotheses about the manifest behavior to be expected. But what exactly is the *place* for content ascriptions within hypothetical explanations?

Explaining a *cognitive phenomenon*, for instance explaining how a subject is able to read other persons' intentions from their gaze behaviour, typically involves putting the cognitive system as a whole within a broader context in which it interacts with certain environmental conditions and with other subjects expressing the gaze behaviour. This is already the case for non-social cognitive phenomena, where the context is constituted by our ability to navigate through a field of cognitive tasks.[14] However, this is even more the case for social cognition: What needs to be explained here are abilities to generate interactive behavior with respect to other subjects initiated by or as a reaction to some physical information input. Explaining behaviors on that level of complexity requires that the concepts that bear the explanatory burden belong to the same sort of level of complexity.[15]

---

[12] According to Mumford, even in those cases the ascription of a dispositio would not be completely void (cf. Mumford 2003, 136f.).

[13] Note that this content depends on the particular cognitive task accomplished in that case. In another case, this type of activity may bear a different content.

[14] Another context would be, in an ecological account of perception, the environment in which an active perceiver is picking up information.

[15] Higher levels of complexity are characterized by the fact that, for each of the states defined on such a level, there exist a multitude of realizing states on some

Thus, when it comes to explaining social cognition, what is required is not only describing how, for instance, electrical or chemical signals are transmitted and further processed by the subject's neural system, rather these physical processes and their properties must be integrated or *bundled* according to some characteristic functional roles for coordinating the behavior of an organism in response to sensory information (cf. Dretske 1988b, Bartels and May 2009), which functional roles would relate to social functions in the case of social cognition. Although it is the physical properties that do the causal work, the components of the mechanism that are *relevant* for the explanation of the phenomenon to be explained are types of physical entities and properties that are individuated by their capacity to fulfill those functional roles the performance of which guarantees the production of the social phenomenon. The physical components of the productive mechanism have to fit exactly the profiles or the patterns of these functional roles. It is important to note that this procedure does not supply the functional roles (= informational contents) with any autonomous causal powers. The job of functional roles lies entirely in the epistemic realm: it consists in providing a sort of filter by which those physical properties fitting the patterns are selected (cf. Bartels and May 2009 for a case from spatial cognition). The explanation is provided by comparably coarse-grained macro-level patterns. Hypotheses have the following form:

> Entities and properties that satisfy functional roles F are able to produce phenomena Φ.

Showing that the physical entities and properties involved actually fulfill these macrolevel patterns, is then a further step which—in our times—can be performed in most cases only rather sketchily.

To summarize, representational explanations in cognitive neuroscience constitute a particular species of mechanistic explanations in a "special science", the species of mechanistic explanations in which the explaining entities and properties are characterized by their informational contents, and in which the mechanism is an information processing mechanism. This reflects a particular explanatory interest:

---

level below. The aspects of systems described by such higher level states generalize over many detailed lower-level states; they are relevant for the 'overall' behavior of a system. An example from physics may help to clarify this point: Concepts like "entropy" in thermodynamics fulfill some autonomous explanatory role by describing the overall behavior of the system in its physical environment—as apart from a fine-grained description of the system based on the interaction of its constituents. For instance, ascribing entropy provides a theoretical description of the behavior of the system within an environment of systems at different temperatures.

the interest of showing how information processing enables the subject to successfully navigate through the physical and social world.

References

Amodio, D.M. and C.D. Frith. 2006. Meeting of minds: the medial frontal cortex and social cognition. *Nature reviews* 7:268–277.

Bartels, A. and M. May. 2009. Functional role theories of representation and content explanation: with a case study from spatial cognition. *Cognitive Processing* 10:63–75.

Bechtel, W. 2001a. The compatibility of complex systems and reduction: A case analysis of memory research. *Minds and Machines* 11:483–502.

Bechtel, W. 2001b. Representations: From neural systems to cognitive systems. In W. Bechtel, P. Mandik, J. Mundale, and R. Stufflebeam, eds., *Philosophy and the Neurosciences. A Reader*, pages 333–348. Blackwell.

Bechtel, W. 2008. *Mental Mechanisms*. Routledge.

Bramham, J., R.G. Morris, J. Hornak, P. Bullock, and C.E. Polkey. 2009. Social and emotional functioning following bilateral and unilateral neurosurgical prefrontal cortex lesions. *Journal of Neuropsychology* 3:125–143.

Charman, T., S. Baron-Cohen, J. Swettenham, G. Baird, A. Cox, and A. Drew. 2000. Testing joint attention, imitation and play as infancy precursors to language and theory of mind. *Cognitive Development* 4:481–498.

Clark, A. 1989. *Microcognition: Philosophy, Cognitive Science and Parallel Distributed Processing*. MIT Press.

Craver, C.F. 2008. Law and mechanistic explanations in the Hodgkin and Huxley model of the action potential. *Philosophy of Science* 75:1022–1033.

Cummins, R. 1975. Functional analysis. *Journal of Philosophy* 72 (20):741–765.

David, N., B. Bewernick, A. Newen, S. Lux, G.R. Fink, N.J. Shah, and K. Vogeley. 2006. The self-other distinction in social cognition–perspective-taking and agency in a virtual ball-tossing game. *Journal of Cognitive Neuroscience* 18:898–910.

David, N., A. Newen, and K. Vogeley. 2008. The "sense of agency" and its underlying cognitive and neural mechanisms. *Consciousness and Cognition* 17:523–534.

Dawson, G., S. Webb, G.D. Schellenberg, S. Dager, S. Friedman, E. Aylward, and T. Richard. 2002. Defining the broader phenotype of autism: genetic, brain, and behavioral perspectives. *Developmental Psychopathology* 3:581–611.

Dretske, F. 1981. *Knowledge and the Flow of Information*. MIT Press.

Dretske, F. 1988a. *Explaining Behavior*. MIT Press.

Dretske, F. 1988b. The explanatory role of content. In R. Grimm and D. Merrill, eds., *Contents of Thought*, pages 31–43. University of Arizona Press.

Frith, C.D. 2007. The social brain? In *Philosophical Transactions of the Royal Society B*, vol. 362, pages 671–678.

Gopnik, A., V. Slaughter, and A.N. Meltzoff. 1994. Changing your views: How understanding visual perception can lead to a new theory of the mind. In C. Lewis and P. Mitchell, eds., *Children's Early Understanding of Mind: Origins and Development*, pages 157–181. Lawrence Erlbaum.

Keyser, C. and V. Gazzola. 2007. Integrating simulation and theory of mind: from self to social cognition. *Trends in Cognitive Science* 11:194–196.

Kuzmanovic, B, A.L. Georgescu, S.B. Eickhoff, N.J. Shah, G. Bente, G.R. Fink, and K. Vogeley. 2009. Duration matters. dissociating neural correlates of detection and evaluation of social gaze. *Neuroimage* 46:1154–1163.

Lieberman, M. 2007. Social cognitive neuroscience: A review of core processes. *Annual Review of Psychology* 58:259–289.

Machamer, P., L. Darden, and C.F. Craver. 2000. Thinking about mechanisms. *Philosophy of Science* 67:1–25.

Mitchell, J.P. 2009. Social psychology as a natural kind. *Trends in Cognitive Science* 13 (6):246–251.

Mumford, S. 2003. *Dispositions*. Clarendon Press.

Mundy, P. 1993. Normal versus high functioning status in autism. *American Journal of Mental Retardation* 97:381–384.

Raichle, M.E., A.M. MacLeod, A.Z. Snyder, W.J. Powers, D.A. Gusnard, and G.L. Shulman. 2001. A default mode of brain function. *Proceedings of the National Academy of Sciences USA* 98:676–682.

Schilbach, L., M. Wilms, S.B. Eickhoff, S. Romanzetti, R. Tepest, G. Bente, N.J. Shah, G.R. Fink, and K. Vogeley. 2010. Minds made for sharing: initiating joint attention recruits reward-related neurocircuitry. *Journal of Cognitive Neuroscience* 22:2702–2715.

Shamay-Tsoory, S.G., R. Tomer, D. Goldsher, B.D. Berger, and J. Aharon-Peretz. 2004. Impairment in cognitive and affective empathy in patients with brain lesions: anatomical and cognitive correlates. *Journal of Clinical and Experimental Neuropsychology* 26:1113–1127.

Tomasello, M., M. Carpenter, J. Call, T. Behne, and H. Moll. 2005. Understanding and sharing intentions: the origins of cultural cognition. *Behavioral and Brain Sciences* 28:675–691.

Vogeley, K., P. Bussfeld, A. Newen, S. Herrmann, F. Happé, P. Falkai, W. Maier, N.J. Shah, G.R. Fink, and K. Zilles. 2001. Mind reading: neural mechanisms of theory of mind and self-perspective. *Neuroimage* 14:170–181.

Vogeley, K., M. May, A. Ritzl, P. Falkai, K. Zilles, and G.R. Fink. 2004. Neural correlates of first-person-perspective as one constituent of human self-consciousness. *Journal of Cognitive Neuroscience* 16:817–827.

Vogeley, K. and A. Roepstorff. 2009. Contextualising culture and social cognition. *Trends in Cognitive Science* 13:511–516.

Woodward, J. 2000. Explanation and invariance in the special sciences. *British Journal for the Philosophy of Science* 51:197–254.

9

Varieties of Representation

Gottfried Vosgerau

Abstract

Philosophical theories of representation often fail to acknowledge that there are two distinctions they have to capture: first, the distinction between non-representations and representations, and second, the distinction between good (successful) representations and poor representations (misrepresentations). I will present and defend a functionalist framework for characterizing representations as opposed to non-representations. The second distinction will be based on specifying adequacy relations holding between the representational vehicles and the represented objects. Within this extended functionalistic framework, misrepresentation can be explained. I will present different adequacy relations that constitute different kinds of representations. After discussing different kinds of representation, I will present some of the advantages of the account, such as the integration of aspects of cognitive development and the interrelations between the account and other ideas within the philosophy of mind.

9.1 Introduction

The word 'representation' can be used in different ways. I will confine it to denote the representational vehicle which represents an object.[1] The represented object is called the *representandum*. The relation between the representandum and the representation will be called the representation relation. Ever since Plato, philosophers tried to describe

---

[1] I use 'object' in the widest sense, i.e., it can be an individual, a property, a state of affairs, an event, or an abstract entity.

Knowledge and Representation.
Albert Newen, Andreas Bartels
& Eva-Maria Jung (eds.).
Copyright © 2011, CSLI Publications.

the representation relation in detail, i.e., to formulate necessary and sufficient conditions for this relation to obtain. Especially in the case of mental representation this matter was and still is heavily discussed.

Theories of representation can be broadly categorized into similarity theories, causal theories, conventional theories, and functionalist theories.[2] They differ in their definition of the representation relation: similarity theories take the relation to be some kind of similarity relation, causal theories state that the representation is caused by the representandum, conventional theories take the relation to be a matter of conventionally established rules, and functionalist theories seek to explain the relation in terms of functions or functional roles of the representation. All of these theories have their characteristic difficulties: similarity theories face the problem of asymmetry of the representation relation, causal theories struggle with the explanation of misrepresentation, conventional theories are implausible for mental representation, and functional theories have to appeal to teleological notions like purpose or interpretation.[3] From these difficulties, some constraints for adequate theories of representation can be inferred: they should be able to explain the asymmetry of the representation relation as well as misrepresentation, they should be equally plausible for mental as well as external representations, and they should avoid to transfer the real problem to other notions like purpose, interpretation, or intention(ality).

Let me begin with the notion of misrepresentation: an entity that does not represent anything is not a misrepresentation but simply no representation at all. A misrepresentation is rather some entity that is used as a representation but fails to be adequate for this purpose. Hence, in order to explain cases of misrepresentation, it is not sufficient to specifiy sufficient and necessary conditions for being a representation, since then we cannot distinguish between good representations and poor representations (misrepresentations). Equally, it is not sufficient to specifiy sufficient and necessary conditions for being a good (successful) representation, since then we cannot distinguish between misrepresentations and entities that are not representations at all. In other words: to specify just one relation as the representation relation is not enough, since one relation either does hold or does not hold and hence splits up the world into two halves. However, we want to have three parts: non-representations, misrepresentations, and good representations.

---

[2]I take teleosemantic theories to be a subclass of functionalist theories.

[3]Due to space limitations, I cannot discuss the different accounts here; for a detailed discussion see Vosgerau (2009b).

The strategy of this paper will be to formulate a revised functionalist theory that specifies necessary and sufficient conditions for being a representation, including good and poor representations. Because a functionalist theory is not able to tell good representations from poor ones,[4] a second relation is then introduced to distinguish among the representations between good and poor ones. This adequacy relation will turn out to be different for different kinds of representations. In this paper, I can only sketch different plausible kinds of representations.

9.2 Functions and Arguments

Functionalism states that the representation relation can be described in terms of the 'function' or the 'functional role' the representation plays for the system. I will start my discussion with a short synopsis of the origins of these notions. I will then develop a new definition of the basic notion of a functional role which leads to a non-teleological functional framework for a theory of representation.

Based on the mathematical theory of abstract automata which describes certain systems on a level that is independent of the physical realization of the system (the implementation), the core idea of functionalism was formulated by Putnam (1975): mental states can be individuated in terms of their functional role alone, independent of their physical realization. The 'behavior' of an automaton can be described by a function mapping the possible states of the automaton and the possible inputs onto the according outputs and subsequent states of the automaton. The states of the automaton play a 'functional role' for the system exactly in the sense that they are arguments of the characteristic function of the system (note that the inputs play functional roles as well). Defining a state via its functional role means that it is characterized only as the argument of a certain function (for which the inputs and outputs are known).

In order to individuate a mental state, it is hence necessary to specify the function of the cognitive system. However, there are differences in which functions are taken into account. Whereas Millikan (1994) takes the relevant functions to be biological (evolutionary) functions, Dretske (1981) seems to have an epistemic function in mind: information can be

---

[4]This critique of functionalism has been debated in the literature; a recent argument to overcome this critique was presented by Bartels and May (2009). However, their argument relies on the assumption that some additional story (which they take to be an integral part of functionalism, but I do not) is able to provide the distinction between good and poor representations, namely "indication functions" and "structural resemblance". In my terminology, these two additions characterize the adequacy relations of representations.

used to gain knowledge.[5] Nevertheless, the representations (the beaver's splashing/the position of the gauge's needle)[6] are arguments of the functions (to survive/to know the amount of fuel) and are thereby mapped onto specific outputs (fleeing behavior/knowledge). The same story applies to mental states, for example the percepts of the splashing and the needle's position. They are arguments of such functions, hence have a functional role. They can be individuated through the specific output they 'generate' (given the input).

Cummins (1989) regards cognitive 'actions' as the relevant functions. In his view, thinking can be viewed as executing functions mapping inputs (knowledge) to outputs (new knowledge). Every mental state has a specific functional role in these cognitive functions. His illustrating example (Cummins 1989, 89f.) is an adding calculator. Its function can be written as $g : \langle C, M, +, N, = \rangle \mapsto D$, where $C, M, +, N, =$ stand for the pushing of the buttons *clear*, *first addend*, *plus*, *second addend*, *equals* and D stands for the display state. Pretty much the same thing applies to the human act of adding: the human mind can be described as performing a function, where the inputs and outputs are mental representations. All of the mental representations as well as the button pushes have their specific functional role and can be individuated just by this role. However, the reason why they are representations of numbers (and mathematical functions) is—according to Cummins— because there is another function 'in the world', namely the adding function $+ : \langle m, n \rangle \mapsto m + n$, and the mental and calculator functions are *interpreted* as representing this function. For mental representation this leads to a dilemma: either I am the one to interpret my own mental representations for which it is necessary to have immediate access to the 'world' function, which would make the representation superfluous, or somebody else is to interpret my mental representations which would mean that they are no longer representations *for me*. The crucial point is that the whole function is taken to represent another function. The single mental states do not represent as such but only in virtue of being arguments of the representing function. I think that Cummins confuses the idea of demonstration[7] or simulation with the notion of representation. The cognitive function may simulate the adding function in a

---

[5] For Dretske, representations have the *function* to carry information, regardless of whether they actually carry it or not.

[6] These are two famous examples for representation from the literature: Millikan's beaver splashing being a representation for danger that makes other beavers flee, and Dretske's position of the gauge's needle representing the amount of fuel in a gas tank.

[7] In the sense introduced by Hughes (1997).

certain way, but it does not represent it, rather, it instantiates it. On the other hand, the mental states do represent numbers, and they do so in virtue of being arguments of the (implementation of the) adding function.

In summary, it seems inappropriate to assume cognitive functions to be the relevant functions for individuating mental representations, since then the representation relation is shifted to the whole function, and therefore some intentional/teleological notion such as interpretation has to be introduced which does not explain the original problem but rather restates it. Much better functions seem to be behavioral and epistemic functions, because they bridge the gap between mind and world (they involve both sides). However, the notion of function must be handled with care: in Dretske's and Millikan's writings the basic idea of functionalism is abandoned to some extend. By introducing a 'function to mean', teleology enters the game. The function to mean is not a function in the mathematical sense, it is rather another expression for being purposefully used to mean. The reason why both theories are ultimately not satisfactory is because the two meanings of the word 'function' are being confused (the mathematical meaning and the meaning of being designed to or being meant to; cf. Vosgerau 2009b).

Teleological notions such as purpose imply a subject of the purpose, i.e., someone who intends a goal. It seems inappropriate for a naturalistic theory of representation to presuppose such a subject, unless the representing subject and the subject of the purpose are the same and the concept of intentionality (in the sense of purpose) is based on the concept of behavior. However, in teleological theories, the representing subject is not the subject of the purpose. In the case of Cummins and Dretske, I cannot be the interpreter of my own mental states because I would need to have direct access to the 'world' function to interpret my representation as representing that function which would make the representation superfluous. Hence, there must be somebody else doing the job. In the case of Millikan's teleosemantics, it is the splashing and ultimately the fleeing behavior that has a function, i.e., that is purposeful. It has acquired this function, namely survival, because of selective processes of evolution. The use of the notion "purpose" should probably be understood as a metaphorical use in this context. As such, it has to be clarified in detail. Moreover, I doubt that an evolutionary explanation will be able to account for an explanation of how representations work: the evolution of fur, for example, can be explained by its function to keep warm (or whatever function it might have). Nevertheless, the explanation of why fur is able to keep animals warm is usually not given (and might even not possibly be given). In the same vein, evolutionary explanations might be able to account for the fact that there are representations, but I doubt that they are able to give fruitful accounts of how these representations work. I will hence avoid teleological notions.

For this purpose, it is appropriate to go back to the original idea based on the mathematical notion of function. As I have already argued above, 'playing a functional role' is to be understood as 'being an argument of some function'. First of all, the relevant types of functions have to be found. A good starting point seems to be behavior.[8] Indeed, behavior can be described as a function mapping some states of affairs onto some new states of affairs. In this sense, the fleeing behavior of the beaver hearing a splashing can be described as a function mapping the actual position of the beaver and the splashing onto a new position of the beaver; the 'behavior' of the model car[9] can be described by a function mapping the right path through the maze and the actual position of the car onto a new position of the car. A functionalist description is not only possible for behavior (or behavior-like events), but also for physical events. The position of the gauge's needle, for example, is a function of the amount of fluid in the tank. Indeed, functionalist descriptions are common in physics: the position of an object is a function of its former position, its impulse, and the forces influencing it; the state of a quantum-mechanical system is described by the so-called 'wave function' mapping states onto states. In this abstract way, all events in the world can be described. Millikan is right that 'function' is a scientific category, but neither do we have to assume the teleological notion nor is it confined to biology. It is up to the empirical sciences such as physics, biology, psychology, sociology, to find the best descriptions for the phenomena. This means that the functions we have to consider are the ones formulated by the sciences.

Intuitively, representations stand for something else, they are proxies.[10] This notion of 'taking the place of something else' is defined in mathematics as substitution: in every function, one argument can be substituted, i.e., replaced, by some other argument. Let us assume that the best description of fleeing behavior of the beaver is given by the

---

[8]Thereby, the famous argument given by Block (1978) is already undermined: the people of China will never behave in the same way as a human for they will never drink *one* cup of tee or go shopping. It is also in this sense that Cummins (1989) is wrong in assuming that cognitive functions are the relevant ones.

[9]Cummins 1996 introduces the example of a model car that navigates through a maze with the help of a moving cogged plastic card with a slit steering the car (cf. Cummins 1996, 93).

[10]This term is borrowed from Cummins (1996).

function f_{FB} : {beaver at x, danger near x} $\mapsto$ beaver at y. This is a general description of the fleeing behavior. However, in the situation where the beaver just hears the splashing of a conspecific, the argument 'danger near x' can be substituted by the splashing:

$$f_{FB}\left[\frac{\text{splashing near } x}{\text{danger near } x}\right] : \{\text{beaver at } x, \text{ splashing near } x\} \mapsto \text{beaver at } y.$$

In this sense, the splashing is a substitute for danger. In Cummins' example of the model car, the right path through the maze can be substituted by the cogged plastic card. In the case of the gauge's needle, the relevant function seems to be an epistemic one, i.e., a function with some kind of knowledge as value. It can be described as a mapping from the amount of fuel onto the knowledge that there is that amount of fuel in the tank. In this function, again, the amount of fuel can be substituted by the position of the needle, yielding the function f_{GN} : position of needle $\mapsto$ knowledge of amount of fuel.

The abstract notion of function is suitable for encompassing the different cases of representation discussed in the literature. This mathematical notion does not involve any teleology or intentionality. It is used in many sciences to describe phenomena and is therefore not an artificial way to talk about events in the world.

My proposal is hence to *define* representations as substitutes in functions which are the best available scientific descriptions of phenomena. This definition has the advantage that it is based on a well-defined and unproblematic mathematical notion, and it also accounts for the basic intuition that representations are 'stand-ins' or 'proxies'. We can now say: a representation represents its representandum because it takes over its functional role. It stands for the represented object.

I assume that for every event there is one function which is characterized by the best (currently available) description.[11] I will call this function the *standard function*, since it is associated with the best description of the event. Under this assumption, my account explains the asymmetry of the representation relation. Every argument that does not occur in the standard function is a representation of the argument for which it is a substitution in the standard function. The standard function of the frog snapping at a fly,[12] for example,

---

[11] There might not be *one* best description, but several best descriptions depending on the purpose of describing. What I have in mind (at least for the case of mental representation) are descriptions that are given by psychophysics, where behavioral reactions are described only in terms of the physical makeup of stimuli. This kind of description has the advantage that it does not assume any function or evolutionary role of the representation at the level of description.

[12] This example is discussed at length by Fodor (1994).

may be f_{FS} : {frog, fly in front of frog} $\mapsto$ fly inside frog. Of course, the frog has to recognize the fly somehow. As we know, it perceives the fly, and this perception ultimately triggers the tongue movement. In this sense, the percept of the frog is a substitute for the fly and hence a representation of it. I further assume that standard functions are formulated by the different sciences, such that it is a task of these sciences to determine the best description. In the case of the frog, for example, Lettvin et al. (1959) famously showed that the frog's percept is probably a substitute only for the position of the fly, for its black color, and for its motion. Therefore, a better description of the event is that the fly with its position and movement is mapped onto a specific tongue movement, such that only these arguments are substituted by the percept. In this way, the function can be specified: $f_{FS'}$: {black dot, position and movement of black dot} $\mapsto$ specific tongue movement. Under this description it is clear that the frog's representation is a black-moving-dot representation rather than a fly representation. Note that the standard functions I introduced do not depend on normal conditions (as is the case for Millikan's 'normal functioning'): Black moving dots are surely not among the normal condition for frogs. (Normal conditions are at most needed in the sense that the frog has to be able to show reactions at all. However, such normal conditions are different from Millikan's in that they do not depend on a previously assumed teleological function of a representation—they are not success conditions.) Nevertheless, the question which description is the best is then not a philosophical question but is to be decided by the relevant sciences.

I propose to regard the substitution in standard functions as a necessary and sufficient condition for representation. Everything that is a substitute is—by definition—a representation.

Definition 1 r represents x iff r is a substitute for x in a standard function .

All the cases discussed in the literature can be explained within this framework. However, an explanation of misrepresentation is not possible, since the distinction between misrepresentations and good representations cannot be made on the grounds of the notions introduced so far. Rather, misrepresentations occur as substitutes in functions as well and hence are just one type of representations. It might be objected that misrepresentations are misrepresentations *because* they cannot fulfill the same functional role as a good representation; thus, they cannot be substitutes in the same functions. The crucial point is how the functions are individuated. If we take functions that describe behavior (as

I do), then the crucial question is how behavior is individuated. There is certainly no easy and straightforward answer to this question. Nevertheless, the following seems to be true: If a representation is not correct, it nevertheless leads to the same (kind of) behavior as a correct representation would have done. If, e.g., the ant misrepresents the location of its nest, it nevertheless shows the same kind of homing behavior (Gallistel 1993) and can thus be described by the same function (cf. Vosgerau et al. 2008a). If we would deny the sameness of behavior in such cases, we would deny the very possibility of behavioral sciences which builds on the principle that cases of misrepresentation (which are evoked by "controlling" factors) lead to the same kind of behavior as correct representations (otherwise, these experimentally evoked cases could not tell us anything about the mechanisms of correct representations).

There are certain types of representations where a sharp dichotomy between misrepresentation and correct representation seems meaningless. Consider, for example, Bohr's famous model of the helium atom. We know that this model is not correct, although it is useful to explain and compute some properties. Hence, we are not ready to call it a misrepresentation. On the other hand, it is, strictly speaking, not a correct representation. There are better representations of the helium atom, and Bohr's model is just not equally good. Nevertheless, it is a representation. Misrepresentations can hence be viewed as the extreme cases of a continuum: they are extremely poor representations. Nevertheless, they are representations just as correct representations are.

In order to specify the degree of adequacy of a representation, a further relation has to be introduced. I will call this further relation the adequacy relation. The basic idea here is that a representation can only take over the functional role of the representandum if it stands in a certain relation to it—intuitively speaking: it has to fit into the function. The criteria for adequacy are, however, not the same for every representation. Therefore, different kinds of representation can be systematically distinguished by their specific adequacy relation. The next sections present a systematic discussion of the varieties of representation.

9.3 Adequacy and the Structure of Representations

A representation is a substitute in a standard function. It is a good representation if it stands in some adequacy relation to its representandum. Cases in which the adequacy relation is not fulfilled are cases of misrepresentation.

Definition 2 r is a misrepresentation of x iff r represents x and r is not adequate in respect to its representing x.[13]

If the adequacy relation allows for varying degrees, there are better and worse representations, depending on the degree to which they are adequate.

Since most theories of representation have not only focused on either the representation relation or the adequacy relation but have also taken specific examples as starting points, the different theories propose widely differing criteria for representations. Moreover, each theory starts with another kind of example and generalizes the relation between the representation and the representandum to all representations.[14] Therefore, all of the theories have a rather limited plausibility when venturing outside their respective starting examples. This effect is due to the fact that there are indeed different adequacy relations, characterizing different kinds of representation.

The functional role, as I defined it, cannot be understood as having a teleological function (a sense). In particular, it stands in a sharp contrast to a 'function to mean' (of the Dretske/Millikan style). It is *not* the function of the representation to be adequate (indeed, I did not talk about any function of the representation). Hence, the functional role does not include or presuppose the adequacy relation. Consider, for example, that you want to grasp an object. You have a mental representation of the position of the object.[15] In one case, this representation is adequate and you succeed in reaching the object. In another case, the position is poorly represented and you fail to reach the object. Nevertheless, both cases are cases of the same kind of behavior, namely object-grasping. Therefore, the function that describes the behavior has to be the same as well. Thus, the functionalist story is the same independent of whether we have a case of successful representation or of misrepresentation. The difference in the two cases is that one representation stands in a certain adequacy relation to the representandum and the other does not.

---

[13]Different adequacy relations are specified below.

[14]For example, Goodman (1976) famously starts with works of art highlighting the conventional aspects of representation; Dretske (1981) discusses the gauge example ending up with a teleosemantic theory based on causal natural meaning; Fodor (1994) analyzes the example of a frog snapping at a fly, thereby stressing the causal component of mental representation; Cummins (1996) chooses the model car example which leads him to propose an isomorphism theory of representation.

[15]It substitutes the position of the object in the function mapping the position of the object and the actual position of your hand onto the new position of your hand.

Indeed, there are different adequacy relations such that different kinds of representations can be defined on the grounds of each specific adequacy relation. I will not argue for every relation in detail, but rather list possible and plausible cases.

9.4 Varieties of Representations

I will first focus on external representations (which are not in the head and can therefore be representations for different people) as opposed to mental representations (which are roughly in the head and can be used only by a single person). I will only sketch the application of the framework to this field and move on to a more in depth discussion of mental representations in Section 9.5 (see also Vosgerau 2009b).

9.4.1 Simple Representations

Let me start with a distinction between simple and complex representations. A complex representation is a representation that is composed out of other representations, whereby the specific combination of those parts contributes to the adequacy of the representation. The word 'frog', for example, consists of different letters standing for different sounds. However, the fact that 'frog' may be used as a representation for a frog has nothing to do with the combination of letters or sounds. Any other combination could be used instead. The word 'frogs', on the contrary, is composed out of the word 'frog' and the morpheme '-s' indicating plural. The fact that 'frogs' usually refers to a plurality of frogs is determined by the composition of its parts. Hence, 'frog' is a simple representation whereas 'frogs' is a complex one.

For external representations, examples of simple representations are the color red representing buildings in maps, letters representing sounds, and some (non-pictographic, non-linguistic) traffic signs representing rules. In all these cases, the relation between the representation and the representandum is made explicit or is explicitly learned. The adequacy relation hence seems to be convention (or definition).

On the other hand, there are simple representations involved in models that are not explicitly defined. Consider, for example, a model of the train stations in a certain city. Even if the single points representing the single stations are not named, we will have no difficulty in finding out which point is representing which station, simply because the connections between the points (the structure) reflect the connections between the stations. Thus, by identifying the different connections that one point has to other points, we can identify the station that is represented by this point. This basic idea is captured by Carnap (1998) (§§ 10–14) with the notion of structural descriptions: if one element is part of a structure $\mathfrak{A}$ that matches another structure $\mathfrak{B}$, it can be identified as representing one specific part of $\mathfrak{B}$ because it shows the same structural dependencies. The relevant adequacy relation for such parts of models may be called structural integration.

Definition 3 r is a simple representation of x iff r represents x and r is not composed of representations such that the composition is relevant for the adequacy relation.

Definition 4 r is a complex representation of x iff r represents x and r is not a simple representation of x.

Definition 5 The adequacy relation for simple representations that are parts of structures is convention or structural integration.

However, this list of simple representations is not exhaustive. Some further examples of simple external representations are given in the next section.

9.4.2 Indices, Icons, and Symbols

The famous distinction of Ch. S. Peirce between indices, icons, and symbols is the first example of how different kinds of representations can be defined on the grounds of different adequacy relations.[16] *Indices* are representations for which the adequacy relation is causality (the representation being caused by the representandum). *Icons*, on the other hand, are representations that are adequate by virtue of some visual resemblance. The adequacy relation for *symbols* is convention.

Although it is far from being clear how conventionalist icons and pictures are,[17] I will not discuss any further whether there are icons in this sense or not.

Definition 6 r is an index of x iff r represents x and r is adequate with respect to its representing x only if it is caused by x.

Definition 7 r is an icon for x iff r represents x and r is adequate with respect to its representing x only if it visually resembles x.

Definition 8 r is a symbol for x iff r represents x and r is adequate with respect to its representing x only if it is conventionally connected to x.

---

[16]The definitions I propose are rough adaptations of the Peircian conception (cf. Peirce 1931) and are not meant to constitute a thorough analysis. Especially, my definition of indices may only constitute a subclass of what Peirce meant with the term.

[17]E.g., Goodman (1976) argued that pictures are fully conventional.

9.4.3 Models

Another type of representations is worth mentioning. Models are not only used, like other kinds of representation, to state something, but also to demonstrate certain relations or mechanisms (cf. Hughes 1997). Therefore, a model must display a structural similarity to the representandum. We can describe both the model and the represented situation as structures in the mathematical sense, i.e., sets over which some functions and/or relations are defined. Structural similarity can be formulated as isomorphism,[18] which holds between two structures $\mathfrak{A}$ and $\mathfrak{B}$ if there is a bijective mapping I between the $a_i \in \mathfrak{A}$ and the $b_i \in \mathfrak{B}$, such that for each function f: $I \left\langle f^{\mathfrak{A}} \left(a_n, a_m, \dots\right)\right\rangle = f^{\mathfrak{B}} \left(b_n, b_m, \dots\right)$ and for every relation R: $R^{\mathfrak{A}} \left(a_n, a_m, \dots\right)$ iff $R^{\mathfrak{B}} \left(b_n, b_m, \dots\right)$.[19]

Most models do not represent the whole structure of the representandum. Bohr's model of atoms, for example, is famous for being restricted to the demonstration of certain phenomena. It is isomorphic to the structure of the Helium atom, but only to a certain degree, i.e., only to a restricted part of it. For this reason, the notion of partial isomorphism is introduced (Bueno 1997, French and Ladyman 1999, French 2002, Bartels 2005). The problem with this notion is that there is always a trivial partial isomorphism[20] between two structures. Therefore, the formal definition does not help as long as a relevant part of the represented structure can be determined. However, depending on the standard function in which the model plays its role there is a relevant part of the representandum's structure. This relevant part is determined by the arguments occurring in the function. Hence, it is only for the represented object that a partial structure must be assumed. This partial structure varies with the functional role of the object.[21] On the side of the representation we must take the whole structure into account. Thus, for a model, the adequacy relation is a partial isomorphism, where the relevant part is determined by the standard function.[22]

---

[18]It is widely discussed whether isomorphism is an appropriate means to describe the representation relation. French (2002) defends the view that isomorphism is necessary and sufficient for models as well as for works of art. Bartels (2005, 2006) presents a general theory of representation that is based on the notion of homomorphism.

[19]Cf. Ebbinghaus et al. (1992), 49.

[20]The same holds for homomorphisms.

[21]Another way of dealing with this problem would be to say that a model does not stand for the whole object but only for the modeled part; I think the common use of 'model' is better matched by the analysis presented here.

[22]See Vosgerau (2006) for a detailed discussion of mental models.

The notion of partial isomorphism allows for varying degrees: a model can be better or worse (for a specific function). Only when it matches the relevant part of the structure exactly, it is a perfect model. If it contains more *or* less elements, relations, or functions, it will be less adequate (although not completely inadequate). In this sense, Bohr's model of the atom is not a misrepresentation, although there are better representations[23] of the same representandum.

Definition 9 r is a model for x iff r represents x and r is adequate in representing x to the degree it is isomorphic to the relevant part of the structure of x, where the relevant part is determined by the arguments taken by the standard function in which x is involved.

9.5 Different Levels of Mental Representation

After having characterized some representations that are shared by humans, I will now proceed to mental representations (which cannot be shared). Mental representations can be divided into four different classes according to four different adequacy relations. This classification parallels different cognitive abilities which are acquired during cognitive development (cf. Newen and Vogeley 2003, Vosgerau et al. 2008b, Vosgerau 2009b).

9.5.1 Sensational Representations

First of all, there are simple mental representations, which are caused by their representandum. If, for example, a light ray causes the cones in the retina to fire, this firing is a mental representation of this light ray, and it is adequate only if it is caused by it. I will call these very basic representations sensational representations, for which the adequacy relation is causality.

Definition 10 r is a sensational representation of x iff r is a mental representation of x, and r is adequate with respect to its representing x only if it is caused by x.

9.5.2 Perceptual Representations

The next step is to combine the sensational representations to form perceptual representations. They are complex, consisting of sensational and/or perceptual representations. The basic idea is that different sensory data have to be integrated in order to perceive something. Following the account of O'Regan and Noë (O'Regan and Noë 2001a,b, Noë 2005), perception means to know the systematic contingencies that

---

[23]Assuming that this function is something like explaining/demonstrating the physics of atoms.

occur with the perceiver's action. To have perceived something, i.e., to classify the input, means to know how the sensory input varies with movements of the perceiver. For example, to perceive a box does involve 'knowledge'[24] about ('skill') how it would look from other directions. In the same vein, perception of the color red consists of 'knowledge' about how the input changes when moving around.[25]

In this approach, perceptual categories are constituted by skills, i.e., they are defined as dispositions. The perceptual skills generate predictions (dependent on our movements) which are used to process the actual input (Helmholtz 1866, von Holst and Mittelstaedt 1950, O'Regan and Noë 2001a, Grush 2004). Constancy effects are illustrating examples of that mechanism: the world does not seem to move when we move our eyes; colors are perceived as uniform and unchanging when we move; objects are not perceived to grow when we get nearer; etc. Perceptual representations can thus be described as predictions that are generated in certain situations by 'perceptual skills'. They are adequate if the prediction is correct, i.e., if they covary with the input given an action. In this way, they represent systematic contingencies between actions and sensory representations. The adequacy relation is thus covariation of the representation with sense input and action. A system equipped with perceptual representations is able to respond to complex stimuli in a differentiated way. It is no longer a detector that merely reacts to one simple stimulus.

Definition 11 r is a perceptual representation of x iff r is a mental representation of x, and r is adequate with respect to its representing x only if it covaries with the systematic contingencies between the representer's actions and the representer's sensory input caused by x.

9.5.3 Conceptual Representations

Perceptual representations consist basically of bundles of properties and actions. They are not object-representations in the full sense, i.e., the object is not represented as such. In other words: the functions in which perceptual representations play their roles take as arguments

---

[24]'Knowledge' here is used in a very weak sense; in my terms it would be simply to have a representation.

[25]This theory of perception is highly controversial (see, e.g., Schlicht and Pompe 2007, Jacob 2006, Vosgerau et al. 2008a). However, due to space limitations I will not discuss the sensorimotor account nor can I discuss whether all representations found in perception are perceptual representations as defined here. There are very good reasons not to think so (e.g., there are conceptual influences in perception), but this approach seems well suited to explain a great deal of relatively basic perceptions. In this sense, the term 'perceptual' for this kind of representation is somewhat misleading; I use it nevertheless due to the lack of a better term.

only properties (and actions), never the object. However, this is required when concepts are involved. To use a concept involves the capacity to attribute a property to an *object*.[26] Therefore, a conceptual representation has to represent the object as distinct from its properties, i.e., there have to be (at least) two analyzable parts in conceptual representations: one that stands for an object and one that stands for a property (Vosgerau 2007). Conceptual representations are thus characterized by an object-property-structure (and nonconceptual representations such as sensational or perceptual representations by the lack of such an object-property-structure).[27]

In the field of human reasoning, the Theory of Mental Models was developed (Johnson-Laird 1983, 2001) to explain human performance in reasoning. The basic idea is that usually situations are modeled in a way such that every object is represented as one object having one or more properties. In this way, Mental Models function very much like external models. Although the Theory of Mental Models is controversial, it highlights the importance of structure-preserving mental representations for reasoning, which can be formalized as being partially isomorphic to the represented situations in the sense presented in Section 9.4.3 (for a detailed discussion of the importance of structure-preservation and its formalization, see Vosgerau 2006). Stenning (2002) argues that Mental Models are not special with respect to isomorphism because it holds for other proposed formats of representation as well; in fact, he shows that Euler Circles, Mental Models, and fragments of natural deduction systems (mental logics) are equivalent.[28] Therefore, I take isomorphism to be the adequacy relation for conceptual representations.

Hence, conceptual representations are complex representations that have analyzable parts which represent objects and analyzable parts that represent properties. The adequacy relation for this type of representation is partial isomorphism. Note, that one crucial feature of conceptual representations is that the generality constraint is fulfilled: if there is a representation for '*a* is *F*' and one for '*b* is *G*', then there exist possible representations '*a* is *G*' and '*b* is *F*' (Evans 1982, 104). Similar

---

[26]I am here assuming the standard interpretation of "concept", as it is also presupposed by the Generality Constraint, the principle of compositionality and systematicity, etc. (see below).

[27]Strictly speaking, not every conceptual representation has to have an object-part, at least not at the surface of its linguistic expression, e.g., "Red is a color". However, every part that figures in such a representation must also figure in representations with proper object-parts.

[28]They all belong to "a family of abstract *individual identification algorithms*" (Stenning and Yule 1997, 109).

constraints can be found in very different accounts of concepts, e.g., in Fodor (1987) (compositionality and systematicity) or in Newen and Bartels (2007) (concepts can be applied to different objects, and one object can by subsumed under different concepts). This ability stems from the structure of the representations and lies at the core of what we call reasoning: inferring new information from given information.

Definition 12 r is a conceptual representation of x iff r is a mental representation of x, and r is adequate in representing x to the degree it is isomorphic to the relevant part of the structure of x, where the relevant part is determined by the arguments taken by the standard function in which x is involved.

The ability to (correctly) represent objects that were never experienced before goes along with the ability to represent non-actual objects. Only systems that have reached the level of (what I call) conceptual representations have the necessary skills to represent objects with which they have no perceptual 'contact'.[29] This involves explicit memories (representing objects that have been experienced before but are no longer being experienced)[30] as well as imagining objects that do not exist. At nonconceptual levels, such representations would be simply misrepresentations, since the adequacy relation is never fulfilled if there is no perceptual 'contact' with the representandum. However, at the conceptual level, the adequacy relation only involves a reference to the structure of objects. Structures are defined mathematically. In this sense, non-actual objects also have such a structure (think of the unicorn having four legs, for example). This structure is an abstract entity and ontologically no more problematic than the natural numbers (which form a structure as well). Therefore, conceptual representations of non-actual objects can be correct and are not automatically misrepresentations (Vosgerau 2008).[31] Some philosophers (e.g., Brentano, Husserl) thought that this characteristic lies at the heart of representation (or aboutness or intentionality, as they sometimes liked to call it). The view presented here clearly differs from this conception in not

---

[29]Newen and Bartels (2007) take this ability even to be part of the definition for conceptual representations.

[30]Note, that this is not a prerequisite for recognition, since recognition does not necessarily involve explicit comparison with other experiences as demonstrated already by the famous PERCEPTRON (Rosenblatt 1958).

[31]This story also applies to fictional objects: we can represent them correctly if we represent their structure which exists as an abstract entity. The structure of a fictional object is defined by the story in which it occurs. In this sense, it is correct to represent that Sherlock Holmes lives in Baker Street. This analysis can be viewed as an extension of the idea of a story-operator introduced by Künne (1983).

taking this point as a mark of representation. My best argument for this is, I think, to have shown that other forms of representation work with the same basic mechanism and yet do not exhibit such characteristics.

9.5.4 Meta-Representations

The highest level of representation is reached with meta-representations. If a system has a meta-representation, then it is not only able to represent a fact p, but also the propositional attitude towards this fact (e.g., 'I believe that p'). Propositional attitudes can be analyzed as functional roles of these representations; hence a meta-representation represents a representation together with its functional role. It does not matter whether this represented functional role is a role for me or for another system. This means that there is no representational difference between 'I believe that p' and 'You believe that p' on the level of their structure.[32] Of course, these meta-representations will have different functional roles.

Ascription of propositional attitudes is associated with explanations and predictions of behavior. We ascribe the wish to eat ice cream to the child in order to explain and predict her behavior. Therefore, a good meta-representation is one that does a satisfactory job, as far as explanation and prediction are concerned. The adequacy relation of meta-representations is therefore explanatory and/or predicting adequacy.[33] Meta-representations enable a system to actively change the way of representing the world and therefore also, the way of interacting with the world. A system at this stage does no longer rely on 'Trial and Error' mechanisms but is able to actively change its own representations in order to produce new behavior (deliberating and planning actions are essentially such productions of new representations). Especially the construction of a so called Theory of Mind, which is a prerequisite for higher social interaction, can take place at this level of representation.[34]

Definition 13 r is a meta-representation of x iff r is mental, r represents x, and r is adequate with respect to its representing x only if it explains and/or predicts the behavior of the bearer of x.

---

[32] The representation of a propositional attitude of somebody else involves the representation of the bearer. In the case of my own attitudes, there may be no such representation of myself involved, at least not an explicit one.

[33] Note that this is true even for so called *de-se*-representations: if I tell you that I really want to quit smoking, you will not believe me unless my behavior is to some degree consistent with the wish expressed (which does not mean that my attempts have to be successful).

[34] For a detailed discussion of meta-representations see Vosgerau (2009c,b).

I presented a framework which can be used to define different types of representation, particularly four types of mental representation. In the remainder of the paper I will present some points in favor of this distinction and mention interrelations to other philosophical theories of mind.

9.6 Outlook and Conclusion

I have presented a functionalist framework for the explanation of representation which specifies necessary and sufficient conditions for being a representation. However, since misrepresentations are also representations, a further relation had to be introduced to distinguish good from poor representations: the adequacy relation. Since there are different adequacy relations, different kinds of representations can be systematically distinguished within this framework. In this outlook, I would like to present some connections with other philosophical debates. The aim of this is not to argue for specific interpretations, but to point to directions in which the presented framework can be (or already has been) applied to other fields.

The philosophical tradition did not pay very much attention to the problem of cognitive development. However, an adequate philosophy of mind should not only be able to describe the normal mental abilities of adults but also make plausible how these abilities can be acquired by a child (cf. Bermúdez 1998). For a naturalist philosophy of mind this means that it should provide an account of cognitive development which is grounded in simple mechanisms and makes plausible the development of higher levels. This claim parallels Chomsky's famous claim that a good linguistic theory should not only describe the rules of a language but also make plausible how these rules can be learned by children. One advantage of the approach to mental representation presented here is that a developmental aspect is already contained. The different levels of mental representation not only logically build on each other but also form a developmental hierarchy. I will briefly present some selected examples of psychological theories of cognitive development and show how they straightforwardly integrate into the proposed framework.

One famous account of cognitive development is formulated by Gibson and Pick (2000). The basic notion introduced is the notion of affordances. Affordances are properties of objects that only exist in relation to a perceiver.[35] Roughly put, they specify what the perceiver can do

---

[35]Of course, affordance theory is discussed very controversially. Especially the claim that affordances, being relational properties, are *directly* perceived, is the cause for many critical discussions. In this paragraph, I do not want to endorse affordance theory but rather show how the general idea can be incorporated into

with the object. For example, a chair has (under normal conditions for a normal adult) the affordance to sit on it. However, the chair has much more such affordances, depending, of course, on the perceiver. In the south of the USA, for example, chairs also have the affordance to be a tool for tossing snakes out of rooms. Affordances are therefore not only dependent on the abilities of the perceiver but also on her habits which are in turn dependent on her environment. Cognitive development can be described in terms of the development of affordances. The affordance of the chair for the toddler, for example, may be an object to climb. As the child's abilities change, the affordances will change as well. As soon as the child learns to walk, she will discover that chairs can be used to pull oneself up or to stand on to reach higher points. The basic idea is that we perceive directly the affordances, and that cognitive development (at least) goes along with the development of perceptual abilities—the more we learn the more we are able to perceive (in terms of affordances). Affordances are special cases of systematic contingencies. To establish such a relation to an object means to learn about the consequences of my own interaction with the object. To learn that climbing on a chair allows me to reach higher points is to learn that, given the object, this action (climbing) systematically results in that change (higher position). The notion of systematic contingencies is much wider: it comprises cases of color perception and the like which are hard to capture in terms of affordances. Consistent with the account presented here, affordances are said to play a role in perception. Affordances are thus straightforwardly interpreted as special kinds of systematic contingencies which are learned when forming a perceptual representation of an object.

The theory of affordances is only apt to handle a quite limited range of mental representations, namely a subclass of what I have called perceptual representations. Halford (1999) presented an account of the development of representation which parallels my proposed levels of mental representation surprisingly well. He introduces seven representational ranks (Halford 1999, 155) reflecting the complexity of representations. Representations of rank 0 are "elemental associations" which are characterized by a simple input-output mapping in a neural network (no hidden layer). They occur in "early infancy" and are basically what I called sensational representations. Representations of rank 1 involve "configural associations", i.e., associations where configurations of features have to be discriminated (not only black vs. white but also

---

the presented framework and thereby hopefully be interpreted in a less controversial way.

black square vs. white square vs. black triangle vs. white triangle). In other words, it is not sufficient just to detect single properties but it is necessary to discover combinations of different features at this stage. Our own movement can be one of these features, of course. Thus, on this level also systematic contingencies (i.e., systematic combinations of own movement patterns and changes in other perceptible features) can be represented. At the level of neuronal networks, this can be achieved by adding a hidden layer.[36] This stage is said to occur between the 4th and the 6th month. At this stage, children "can represent perceptible features, but presumably have no explicit representations of relations" (Halford 1999, 156). Therefore, the specification of rank 1 representations nicely fits with my description of perceptual representations. Rank 2 through rank 6 representations can deal with relations, where rank 2 representations deal with unary relations of the structure 'Predicate(Argument)', rank 3 representations with binary relations of the structure 'Predicate(Argument1,Argument2)', and so on until rank 6 representations dealing with quinary relations. Since in these kinds of representation a clear difference is made between objects and their properties, these stages directly correspond to conceptual representations (where no further distinction is made between differences in the complexity of the represented relations). Rank 2 representations occur at the age of 1 year already and rank 6 are likely not to occur in most adults. Neural networks can be specified for each of the ranks (for details see Halford 1999, 158f.).

However, there is no equivalent of meta-representations in Halford's account, although there is an overwhelming amount of research in this field, starting with the classical False-Belief-Task of Wimmer and Perner (1983), which reliably shows that children acquire meta-representations around the age of 4 years. This kind of representation presupposes that features of representations can be represented. One possibility to realize this kind of representation in neural networks could be to 'forward' the representation in one network to another network which then classifies the representation, i.e., which represents the functional role (a property) of the representation.

Besides cognitive development, the functionalist framework I presented incorporates the widespread idea of 'embedded cognition', since the relevant functions take as arguments both objects in the world and the behavior of a cognitive system. In this sense, representation is defined only for creatures that are embedded in an environment. The fact

---

[36]In fact, these neuronal networks do nothing else than 'registering' systematic contingencies of the input.

that behavior is part of the relevant functions takes into account the idea of 'embodied cognition', i.e., the idea that mental representations essentially depend on the cognitive system's body interacting with the environment. Since the relevant functions include behavior, and behavior is essentially involving the body, this general idea finds its place in the proposed framework as well. However, the notion 'mental' was used here quite intuitively: the idea behind it is that a representation is external if it can be used by different cognitive systems and otherwise, it is internal or mental. However, due to space limitations the debate about vehicle externalism (Clark and Chalmers 1998) cannot be taken on here. Nevertheless, the intuitive way of using 'mental' should suffice for the present purpose since important differences between internal and external representations can be specified (e.g., internal representations cannot be symbols) independently of the question whether the term 'mental' refers to things outside our skulls or not.

The account of representations given here can be fruitfully applied to different kinds of problems. For example, a theory of self-consciousness that builds on the levels of mental representation is able to explain the specific direct self-relation of self-conscious states as well as high-level phenomena such as the judgment of authorship for the own thoughts (Vosgerau and Newen 2007, Vosgerau 2009b). In particular, the account is able to give a detailed analysis of psychiatric disorders concerning self-consciousness (Synofzik et al. 2008b,a, Vosgerau 2009a) as well as a new analysis of features of linguistic self-ascription and the underlying I-thoughts (Vosgerau 2009c). Also, the level-theory of self-representation provides new accounts of the cultural dependence of self-construals (Schlicht et al. 2009) and for the understanding and characterization of emotions (Zinck and Newen 2008). Moreover, it has been applied to shed new light on the different formats of spatial representation (Vosgerau 2007). However, the phenomenal quality of our experiences can be shown not to be grounded in special kinds of representations or representational contents, i.e., there cannot be such a thing as 'phenomenal content' (Vosgerau et al. 2008a). Rather, the only possible explanation of phenomenality is based on the idea that the processing of mental representations is responsible for whether they enter into phenomenal consciousness or not.

Acknowledgements

I would like to thank Albert Newen for endless discussions as well as one anonymous reviewer for very helpful comments.

References

Bartels, A. 2005. *Strukturale Repräsentation*. mentis.

Bartels, A. 2006. Defending the structuralist concept of representation. *Theoria* 55:55–67.

Bartels, A. and M. May. 2009. Functional role theories of representation and content explanation: with a case study from spatial cognition. *Cognitive Processing* 10:63–75.

Bermúdez, J.L. 1998. *The Paradox of Self-Consciousness*. The MIT Press.

Block, N. 1978. Troubles with functionalism. In C. Savage, ed., *Perception and Cognition: Issues in the Foundation of Psychology*, vol. IX of *Minnesota Studies in the Philosophy of Science*, pages 261–325. University of Minnesota Press.

Bueno, O. 1997. Empirical adequacy: A partial structures approach. *Studies in History and Philosophy of Science* 28:585–610.

Carnap, R. 1998. *Der logische Aufbau der Welt*. Felix Meiner Verlag, 2nd edn.

Clark, A. and D. Chalmers. 1998. The extended mind. *Analysis* 58 (1):7–19.

Cummins, R. 1989. *Meaning and Mental Representation*. The MIT Press.

Cummins, R. 1996. *Representations, Targets, and Attitudes*. The MIT Press.

Dretske, F. 1981. *Knowledge and the Flow of Information*. Basil Blackwell.

Ebbinghaus, H.-D., J. Flum, and W. Thomas. 1992. *Einführung in die mathematische Logik*. [english translation: 1994. *Mathematical Logic*. Springer.]: BI-Wissenschaftsverlag.

Evans, G. 1982. *The Varieties of Reference*. Oxford University Press.

Fodor, J. 1987. *Psychosemantics*. The MIT Press.

Fodor, J. 1994. Fodor's guide to mental representation. In S. Stich, ed., *Mental Representation. A Reader*, pages 9–33. Blackwell.

French, S. 2002. A model-theoretic account of representation. *Proceedings of the PSA* Supplement.

French, S. and J. Ladyman. 1999. Reinflating the semantic approach. *International Studies in the Philosophy of Science* 13:99–117.

Gallistel, C.R. 1993. *The Organization of Learning*. The MIT Press.

Gibson, E. J. and A. D. Pick. 2000. *An Ecological Approach to Perceptual Learning and Development*. Oxford University Press.

Goodman, N. 1976. *Languages of Art*. Hackett Publishing Company.

Grush, R. 2004. The emulation theory of representation: Motor control, imagery, and perception. *Behavioral and Brain Sciences* 27:377–442.

Halford, G.S. 1999. The properties of representations used in higher cognitive processes: Developmental implications. In I. Sigel, ed., *Development of Mental Representation*, pages 147–168. Lawrence Erlbaum Associates.

Helmholtz, H. 1866. *Handbuch der Physiologischen Optik*. Voss.

Hughes, R.I.G. 1997. Models and representation. *Philosophy of Science (Proceedings)* 64:325–336.

Jacob, P. 2006. Why visual experience is likely to resist being enacted. *Psyche* 12:1–12.

Johnson-Laird, P.N. 1983. *Mental Models.* Harvard University Press.

Johnson-Laird, P.N. 2001. Mental models and deduction. *Trends in Cognitive Sciences* 5 (10):434–442.

Künne, W. 1983. *Abstrakte Gegenstände. Semantik und Ontologie.* Suhrkamp.

Lettvin, J.Y., H.R. Maturana, W.S. McCulloch, and W.H. Pitts. 1959. What the frog's eye tells the frog's brain. *Proceedings of the IRE* 47 (11):1940–1951.

Millikan, R.G. 1994. Biosemantics. In S. Stich, ed., *Mental Representation. A Reader*, pages 243–258. Blackwell.

Newen, A. and A. Bartels. 2007. Animal minds and the possession of concepts. *Philosophical Psychology* 20:283–308.

Newen, A. and K. Vogeley. 2003. Self-representation: Searching for a neural signature of self-consciousness. *Consciousness and Cognition* 12:529–543.

Noë, A. 2005. *Action in Perception.* Cambridge MA, London: MIT Press.

O'Regan, J.K. and A. Noë. 2001a. A sensorimotor account of vision and visual consciousness. *Behavioral and Brain Sciences* 22:939–973.

O'Regan, J.K. and A. Noë. 2001b. What it is like to see: A sensorimotor account of vision and visual consciousness. *Synthese* 192:79–103.

Peirce, C.S. 1931. *Collected papers of Charles Sanders Peirce.* Harvard University Press. Edited by Charles Hartshorne and Paul Weiss.

Putnam, H. 1975. The nature of mental states. In *Mind, language, and reality*, pages 429–440. Cambridge University Press.

Rosenblatt, F. 1958. The perceptron: A probabilistic model for information storage in the brain. *Psychological Review* 65:386–408.

Schlicht, T. and U. Pompe. 2007. Rezension von Alva Noë: Action in Perception. *Zeitschrift für philosophische Forschung* 61:250–254.

Schlicht, T., A. Springer, K.G. Volz, G. Vosgerau, M. Schmidt-Daffy, D. Simon, and A. Zinck. 2009. Self as a cultural construct? An argument for levels of self-representation. *Philosophical Psychology* 22:687–709.

Stenning, K. 2002. *Seeing Reason.* Oxford University Press.

Stenning, K. and P. Yule. 1997. Image and language in human reasoning: A syllogistic illustration. *Cognitive Psychology* 34:109–159.

Synofzik, M., G. Vosgerau, and A. Newen. 2008a. Beyond the comparator model: A multifactorial two-step account of agency. *Consciousness and Cognition* 17:219–239.

Synofzik, M., G. Vosgerau, and A. Newen. 2008b. I move, therefore I am: A new theoretical framework to investigate agency and ownership. *Consciousness and Cognition* 17:411–424.

von Holst, E. and H. Mittelstaedt. 1950. Das Reafferenzprinzip. *Die Naturwissenschaften* 20:464–476.

Vosgerau, G. 2006. The perceptual nature of mental models. In C. Held, M. Knauff, and G. Vosgerau, eds., *Mental Models and the Mind: Current Developments in Cognitive Psychology, Neuroscience, and Philosophy of Mind*, Advances in Psychology, pages 255–275. Elsevier.

Vosgerau, G. 2007. Conceptuality in spatial representation. *Philosophical Psychology* 20:349–365.

Vosgerau, G. 2008. Adäquatheit und Arten mentaler Repräsentationen. *Facta Philosophica* 10:67–82.

Vosgerau, G. 2009a. Die Stufentheorie des Selbstbewusstseins und ihre Implikationen für das Verständnis psychiatrischer Störungen. *Journal für Philosophie und Psychiatrie* 2 (2).

Vosgerau, G. 2009b. *Mental Representation and Self-Consciousness. From Basic Self-Representation to Self-Related Cognition.* mentis.

Vosgerau, G. 2009c. Stufen des Selbstbewusstseins: Eine Analyse von Ich-Gedanken. *Grazer Philosophische Studien* 78:101–130.

Vosgerau, G. and A. Newen. 2007. Thoughts, motor actions, and the self. *Mind & Language* 22 (1):22–43.

Vosgerau, G., T. Schlicht, and A. Newen. 2008a. Orthogonality of phenomenality and content. *American Philosophical Quarterly* 45:309–328.

Vosgerau, G., T. Schlicht, A. Springer, and K.G. Volz. 2008b. Kulturabhängigkeit in einer Stufen-Theorie der Selbst-Repräsentation. In K. Vogeley, T. Fuchs, and M. Heinze, eds., *Psyche zwischen Natur und Kultur*, pages 177–197. Parodos & Pabst Science Publishers.

Wimmer, H. and J. Perner. 1983. Beliefs about beliefs: Representation and constraining functions of wrong beliefs in young children's understanding of deception. *Cognition* 13:103–128.

Zinck, A. and A. Newen. 2008. Classifying emotion: A developmental account. *Synthese* 161:1–25.

10

Why Cognitive Neuroscience Should Adopt a "Pragmatic Stance"

Andreas K. Engel

10.1 Introduction

In the cognitive sciences, we currently witness a "pragmatic turn"[1] away from the traditional representation-centered framework towards a paradigm that focusses on understanding the intimate relation between cognition and action. Such an "action-oriented" paradigm has earliest and most explicitly been developed in robotics, and has only recently begun to gain impact on cognitive psychology and neurobiology. The basic concept is that cognition should not be understood as a capacity of deriving world-models, which then might provide a "database" for thinking, planning and problem-solving. Rather, it is emphasized that cognitive processes are not only closely intertwined with action but that cognition can actually best be understood as "enactive", as a form of practice itself. Cognition, on this account, is grounded in a

---

[1]The term "pragmatic" is used here to make reference to action-oriented viewpoints such as those developed by the founders of philosophical pragmatism, William James, Charles Sanders Peirce or John Dewey. Grossly simplifying, pragmatism entails, for instance, that an ideology or proposition is true if it works satisfactorily, that the meaning of a proposition is to be found in the practical consequences of accepting it, and that unpractical ideas are to be rejected. However, using the term "pragmatic turn", I do *not* mean to suggest a return to exactly the positions put forward by these authors.

Knowledge and Representation.
Albert Newen, Andreas Bartels
& Eva-Maria Jung (eds.).
Copyright © 2011, CSLI Publications.

pre-rational understanding of the world that is based on the sensorimotor exploration of real-life situations.

The goal of this chapter is to discuss possible implications of this
"pragmatic turn" for cognitive neuroscience. I will first summarize, with
a focus on vision research, key assumptions of the classical cognitivist
framework. Subsequently, I will outline the alternative view that results
from the pragmatic turn, and briefly discuss sources and proponents of
this view. In addition to reviewing major conceptual components of this
new framework, I will discuss neurobiological evidence in support of this
notion. As I will argue, new vistas on the "meaning", the functional
roles and the presumed "representational" nature of neural processes
are likely to emerge from this confrontation.

10.2 The Classical Framework of Cognitive Science

Numerous authors have criticized the "orthodox" stance of cognitive
science[2] and, hence, I confine myself to a brief summary of the essential
features. In a nutshell, the following core assumptions characterize the
classical cognitivist view:

- Cognition is understood as computation over representations.[3]
- The subject is conceived as a detached observer with a "bird's eye"
  view on the world.
- Intentionality is explained by the representational nature of mental
  states.
- The architecture of cognitive systems is conceived as being largely
  modular and the functioning of system components is considered as
  strongly context-invariant.
- Computations are thought to be independent of their substrate.
- Explanatory strategies typically refer to inner states of individual
  cognitive systems.

These assumptions, which go back to the work of Fodor (1987, 1990),
Newell and Simon (1976), Fodor and Pylyshyn (1988), Rey (1997)
and other protagonists of the computational/representational theory
of mind, seem to be present, albeit with different emphasis, in all versions and schools of cognitivist theorizing.

---

[2]See, for example, Winograd and Flores (1986), Varela et al. (1991), Chapman
(1991), Dreyfus (1992), Kurthen (1992, 1994), Agre (1997), Clancey (1997), Clark
(1997, 1999, 2008), Engel and König (1998), O'Regan and Noë (2001), Noë (2004,
2009).

[3]Discussing the notion of "representation" is clearly beyond the scope of this
chapter. What I broadly refer to is the concept as used in the Representational
Theory of Mind, see below.

In the following, I will briefly consider theories on visual perception, many of which have been built on the basis of the representational theory of mind. These include, for instance, Marr's theory of vision (cf. Marr 1982) or Biederman's theory of "recognition-by-components" (cf. Biederman 1987). Both of these approaches can be characterized as attempts to develop a theory of "pure vision" (Churchland et al. 1994, Engel and König 1998), that is, an account that tries to explain visual processing in isolation, largely ignoring the relevance that the system dynamics at large, the body or the environment might have for understanding what is meant by "seeing".

Clearly, a key feature of these cognitivist theories of vision is a representational account of perception. Perception is essentially conceived as a "homomorphic mapping" from the external world onto internal states of the cognitive system. This mapping is supposed to preserve structural relations, i.e., constituents of the representation "stand in" for parts of the represented object (cf. Palmer 1999). Vision, on this account, consists in recovering features of a pre-given world, and construction of internal images that, in their entirety, make up a "world-model". The world model serves as a database containing general-purpose knowledge about the external world in the format of explicit and largely context-invariant object descriptions, which are formed independently of situational context or current action. Aloimonos and Rosenfeld (1991) summarize this view by stating:

> Regarding the central goal of vision as scene recovery makes sense. If we are able to create, using vision, an accurate representation of the three-dimensional world and its properties, then using this information we can perform any visual task. (Aloimonos and Rosenfeld 1991, 1250)[4]

In a well-known textbook, Churchland and Sejnowski have aptly coined the slogan "Brains are world-modelers" (Churchland and Sejnowksi 1992, 143).

Obviously, the advocates of this view subscribe to epistemological realism, i.e., they consider the world as existing independent of and prior to any cognitive activity. The world "out there" is conceived as a universe of independent and context-free physical entities, which are all neutral with respect to the cognitive agent who might enter the scene. In the vision theories referred to above, such an "object ontology" can clearly be identified as part of the conceptual framework. As one conse-

---

[4]It should be mentioned that Aloimonos and Rosenfeld, while reviewing the computer vision paradigm of "scene recovery", at the end of their article consider a new paradigm which they call "purposive vision"; showing some similarity to the view advocated here, this paradigm shifts the focus to vision-guided behavior.

TABLE 1
Fundamental stances of "orthodox" cognitive science.

Reductionism	Mental states caused by neural processes; privileged role of neurophysiological models
Representationalism	Cognition as world-modelling
Computationalism	Dominance of the computer metaphor
Atomism	Modular organization of processing
Individualism	Focus on inner states of the cognitive system

quence, early theories on perceptual segmentation have assumed that natural scenes have objectively defined boundaries or predetermined "breaking points", that is, there is only one "correct" way of breaking down a scene into meaningful chunks of information. In this framework, the task of a sensory system is merely to find the correct solution to the segmentation problem (cf. Marr 1982, Biederman 1987).

Both conceptually and methodologically, "atomism" has also played a leading part on the stage of the cognitivist drama. A pervasive assumption was that of modularity—the notion of independent processing systems. Applied to vision theory, the idea prevailed that the visual modality might operate independently of other sensory modalities, of previous learning, goals, motor planning or motor execution. Vision, thus, was assumed to build a purely eidetic world model, supplied to other subsystems only at a late stage:

> The assumption is that the visual system consists of a number of modules that can be studied more or less independently. [...] The integration of modules is assumed to be primarily 'late' in nature" (Ullman 1991, 310).

Cast into a research strategy that dominated the field in the decades, roughly, between 1960 and 1990, this inspired attempts to study effects of isolated stimuli on neuronal responses and to focus on the single cell as most relevant for psychological (*sic!*) description (cf. Barlow 1972, Hubel 1988). In a seminal paper, Barlow expressed the belief that "[i]t no longer seems completely unrealistic to attempt to understand perception at the atomic single-unit level" (Barlow 1972, 382). As a sibling to atomism, individualism (cf. Burge 1979) also dominated the field, and it seemed appropriate to approach cognition with a "tunnel view" focussing exclusively on the inner states of cognitive systems.

10.3   Criticizing Orthodoxy

Several decades further down the road, looking back on the apparently limited success of cognitivist science, it seems hard to escape scepticism: Does such a "theory of pure vision" suffice to establish an adequate account of perception? Do the basic conceptual and methodological premises provide an adequate background? I will argue that they do not—and thus, it's time for a change! I do not want to critically examine each of the assumptions of the orthodox framework in detail, since this has been the subject of numerous masterly writings (e.g., Winograd and Flores 1986, Varela et al. 1991, Dreyfus 1992, Kurthen 1992, Clark 1997). A few remarks may suffice before I move on to describing what might be considered an alternative.

A key question in the debate is whether the representational account adequately describes the nature of cognition, and the relation between cognitive system and world. As stated above, the representational theory of mind implies (i) realism: perceptually relevant distinctions are "fixed" and observer-independent; (ii) a separation of cognitive system and world: the subject is conceived as a detached observer who is not "engaged in" the world; and (iii) passivity of the cognitive system which behaves in a merely receptive way, just "re"-acts, and takes copies of prespecified information. Along all these lines, I suggest, the orthodox stance misconstrues the relation between cognitive system and world, and it actually fails to appreciate the very nature of cognitive processes. In the following, I will highlight some intuitions that raise discomfort with the orthodoxy.

Long before the emergence of research on "active vision" (Findlay and Gilchrist 2003), philosophers have emphasized the active nature of perception. The American pragmatist John Dewey stated:

> Upon analysis, we find that we begin not with a sensory stimulus, but with a sensori-motor coordination, [...] and that in a certain sense it is the movement which is primary, and the sensation which is secondary, the movement of the body, head and eye muscles determining the quality of what is experienced. In other words, the real beginning is with the act of seeing; it is looking, and not a sensation of light [...]. (Dewey 1896, 358–359)[5]

With striking convergence, the same thought can be found more than 40 years later in the writings of the French phenomenologist Merleau-Ponty who concluded that

---

[5]Note the striking resemblance between the notion of "sensori-motor coordination" used by Dewey and the concept of "sensori-motor contingencies" introduced by O'Regan and Noë (2001).

[t]he organism cannot properly be compared to a keyboard on which the external stimuli would play [...]. Since all the movements of the organism are always conditioned by external influences, one can, if one wishes, readily treat behaviour as an effect of the milieu. But in the same way, since all the stimulations which the organism receives have in turn been possible only by its preceding movements which have culminated in exposing the receptor organ to external influences, one could also say that behavior is the first cause of all stimulations. Thus the form of the excitant is created by the organism itself [...]. (Merleau-Ponty 1962, 13)

Perception, according to these authors, is a constructive process whose operations are highly selective. Perceptual acts define, first of all, relevant distinctions in the field of sensory experience, and this occurs by virtue of the cognitive system's neural and bodily organization, as well as "top-down" factors (cf. Engel et al. 2001) such as previous learning, emotion, expectation or attention. Perception, on this account, is not neutral with respect to action, but arises from sensorimotor couplings by which the cognitive agent engages in the world (cf. Varela et al. 1991, O'Regan and Noë 2001). Eventually, this overturns the central notions of the representational theory of mind: the purpose of sensory processing is the guidance of action, not the formation of mental representations.

10.4   The Concept of a Pragmatic Turn

The "pragmatic" stance can be seen as a direct antagonist of the cognitivist framework, implicating a point-by-point opposing view regarding each of the assumptions that have been discussed above:

- Cognition is understood as a capacity of generating structure by action.[6]
- The cognitive agent is immersed in the task domain.

[6]The concept of "action" contrasts with that of "behaviour" and also with that of "movement". Evidently, there are many instances of action which do not involve any (overt) movement. Mental calculation would be a case in point. Conversely, movement does not always imply performance of an "act" (e.g in the case of reflexes). The description of "acts" or "actions" typically makes reference to goals, that often the agent has adopted on the basis of an overall practical assessment of his options and opportunities. "Acts" require plans and decisions, and they typically can be refrained from. "Behavior", in contrast, can be described and explained (at least according to certain psychological schools) without making reference to mental events or to internal psychological processes. Clearly, therefore, the pragmatic turn does not lead back to "behaviorism".

- System states acquire meaning by their functional role[7] in the context of action.
- The architecture of cognitive systems is conceived as being dynamic, context-sensitive and captured best by holistic approaches.
- The functioning of cognitive systems is thought to be inseparable from its substrate or incarnation ("embodiment").
- Explanations make reference to agent-environment or agent-agent-interactions ("situatedness").

Clearly, it's time for a turn, and the central credo of the proponents of the new paradigm could be phrased as "cognition is action" (cf. Varela et al. 1991, Kurthen 1992). That said, the adherents of this motto are facing challenges that may be even more severe than the ones discussed for the cognitivist legacy above. Obviously, the pragmatic credo needs both explication and elaboration. It needs to be spelled out what the implications of this view might be, and whether it has the potential to inspire a new style of thinking or, even more importantly, new styles of designing and performing experiments.

The pragmatic turn, as envisaged here, is rooted in European and American philosophical movements of the late 19th and early 20th century. Tracing these roots would require a detailed analysis that is far beyond the scope of this chapter, and only few remarks will be made to highlight some of the important links. On the one hand, American pragmatism has been influential, with John Dewey (1859-1952) and George Herbert Mead (1863-1931) as two leading protagonists. Dewey's early sensorimotor approach to perception has been cited already (cf. Dewey 1896), and many aspects developed in later writings such as his "event ontology" and his genetic analysis of mind as emerging from cooperative activity (cf. Dewey 1925) are highly relevant in this context. In a similar vein, Mead's theory of the emergence of mind and self from the interaction of organic individuals in a social matrix (cf. Mead 1934) and his analysis of perception and the constitution of reality as a field of situations through the "act" (cf. Mead 1938) bear high relevance to pragmatic cognitive science and deserve further exploitation.

On the other hand, there are clear and explicit links to the European phenomenological-hermeneutic tradition, notably, to the early writings of Martin Heidegger (1889-1976) and the writings of Maurice Merleau-Ponty (1908-1961). Essentially all motives of the pragmatic turn can

---

[7]The notion of "functional role" is also employed in "functional role theories" of representation (e.g., Cummins 1996). However, Cummins seems to consider primarily the system-internal functional role of a mental state which lies in its capacity to affect other mental states (cf. Bartels and May 2009), rather than emphasizing a role in the generation of action.

be traced back to these two philosophers,[8] as noted by proponents of this new view (cf. Dreyfus 1992, Varela et al. 1991, Kurthen 1992, 1994, Clark 1997, Noë 2004). As cited above already, Merleau-Ponty strongly advocated an anti-representationalist view, emphasizing that the structures of the perceptual world are inseparable from the cognitive agent (cf. Merleau-Ponty 1962, 1963) and that, therefore, "world-making" rather than "world-mirroring" lies at the heart of cognition. Heidegger developed his concept of "being-in-the-world" ("*In-der-Welt-Sein*", adopted by Merlau-Ponty using the expression of "*être-au-monde*") to overcome the Cartesian split between subject and world and to ground intentionality (cf. Heidegger 1986, 1989). From this new way of conceiving the relation between subject and world, characterized by mutual intertwinement, a direct path leads to a redefinition of the cognitive system as an "extended mind", including both the cognitive agent and its environmental niche (cf. Varela et al. 1991, Kurthen 1992, 1994, Clark 1997, 2008). The relation to the world can only be one that is rooted in practice, in acting; and practice, in turn, is mediated through the body. Thus, both Merleau-Ponty and Heidegger develop a view of cognition as grounded in concrete sensorimotor activity, in a pre-rational practical understanding of the world (cf. Heidegger 1986, 1989, Merleau-Ponty 1962, 1963). From these premises, two concepts unfold which are of key importance to pragmatic cognitive science: the concept of "situation" (or "situatedness") and the concept of "embodiment".

According to Heidegger and Merleau-Ponty, what we encounter as cognitive agents are never "bare" objects or arrays of contingent features but, rather, meaningful situations, i.e., contexts which we have already structured by prior activity and in which objects are defined as a function of our needs and concerns. Even for the newborn, the world is not a heap of coincident features, since its own needs in concert with the social context define what the world should look like. In his phenomenological analysis of situatedness, Heidegger coins the term "*Bewandtnisganzheit*" (cf. Heidegger 1989), denoting a "referential nexus" across all components of the situation which is, thus, characterized by a holistic structure, and a merging or "intertwinement" of cognitive system and world. Building upon Heidegger's and Merleau-Ponty's insights, Dreyfus pointed out that

> [a] normal person experiences the objects of the world as already interrelated and full of meaning. There is no justification for the assumption

---

[8]Actually, the route these concepts have taken from phenomenology to cognitive science has, in part, led through robotics (cf. Dreyfus 1992, Winograd and Flores 1986, Brooks 1991, Chapman 1991, Agre 1997).

that we first experience isolated facts, [...] and then give them significance. (Dreyfus 1992, 269-270)

Criticizing the ontological assumptions of classical artificial intelligence research, he emphasized that

> [t]he situation is organized from the start in terms of human needs and propensities which give the facts meaning, make the facts what they are, so there is never a question of storing and sorting through an enormous list of meaningless, isolated data. (Dreyfus 1992, 262)

As part of the pragmatic view advocated here, these considerations suggest that the cognitivist ontology of "neutral features" should be replaced by a holistic[9] ontological framework. Following Merleau-Ponty, the world does not have a pre-specified structure that exists prior to, and independent of, any cognitive activity. Rather, the world is an *a-priori* unlabelled "field of experience" where cognition (as embodied action) draws relevant distinctions. If indeed the world is organized in "referential wholes" that cannot be decomposed into neutral objects, then the concept of "situation" should figure as the more basic ontological category.

Clark (1997) has discussed a number of consequences arising from this view. "Situatedness", on his view, implies that cognition does not build upon universal, context-invariant models of the world, but is subject to constraints of the local spatiotemporal environment which need to be coped with in a highly context-dependent manner. This leads Clark to a notion of "minimal representationalism" that posits "action-oriented representations". This denotes the idea that internal states simultaneously describe aspects of the world and "prescribe" possible actions—a view that for him provides a compromise between the cognitivist and the pragmatic framework.

Furthermore, Clark uses the concepts of situatedness and embeddedness to counteract the individualist stance of cognitivism. These notions imply a fundamental coupling through the ongoing interaction between cognitive agent and environment. Therefore, the latter should not be viewed only as a task domain, but also as a resource that "scaffolds" cognitive acts. Slightly radicalizing this insight, one might then say that, in fact, the cognitive system comprises the brain, the body, and the environment (cf. Kurthen 1992, 1994, 2007). As Clark phrases it:

---

[9]Using the term "holism" I refer to the view that the phenomena relevant to a theory of cognition cannot be understood or predicted by studying lower-level elements in isolation, because the significance of the latter depends crucially on the context they are embedded in.

[I]n the light of all this, it may [...] be wise to consider the intelligent system as a spatio-temporally extended process not limited by the tenuous envelope of skin and skull. [...] Cognitive science [...] can no longer afford the individualistic, isolationist biases that characterized its early decades. (Clark 1997, 221)

Summarizing this part of the discussion, I conclude that the concept of situatedness might help to overcome the cognitivist misconstrual of the agent-world relationship, to modify ontological assumptions, and overcome the limitations of an individualist-reductionist approach. As I will discuss in the next section of this chapter, this approach may also change much of our general perspective on the brain's functional architecture and our view on the significance of internal states.

Compared to Clark (1995, 1997, 1999), other eminent proponents of the pragmatic turn, such as Varela, O'Regan, Noë or Kurthen share a more radical rejection of the cognitivist view (cf. Varela et al. 1991, O'Regan and Noë 2001, Kurthen 1992, 1994, 2007). Drawing on the phenomenological tradition, Varela et al. (1991) have explored the implications of defining "cognition as embodied action" (172). As they emphasize, cognition should be considered from the viewpoint of action. Cognition is not detached contemplation, but a set of processes that determine possible actions. Perception, accordingly, must be understood as a process of defining relevant boundaries, not of grasping pre-existing features, and "perceiving a world" means distinguishing possibilities for action. The criterion for success of cognitive operations is not a "veridical representation" of environmental features, but viable action in a given situation.—In a nutshell, cognition, as Varela puts it, can be understood as the capacity of "enacting" a world:

> The overall concern of the enactive approach to perception is not to determine how some perceiver-independent world is to be recovered; it is, rather, to determine the common principles or lawful linkages between sensory and motor systems that explain how action can be perceptually guided in a perceiver-dependent world. (Varela et al. 1991, 173)

> Consequently, cognition is no longer seen as problem solving on the basis of representations; instead, cognition in its most encompassing sense consists in the enactment or bringing forth of a world by a viable history of structural coupling. (Varela et al. 1991, 205)

Exploiting Heideggerian thinking, Kurthen (1992, 1994, 2007) has developed a "hermeneutical theory of cognition". The term "hermeneutic", in his account, is not referring to a hermeneutic nature of the scientific method, but rather to the idea that cognition itself is construed as a hermeneutical faculty. In his framework,

[i]ntentionality is not generated by representation, but [...] by primarily non-representational concrete activity of the cognitive system within its environmental niche. (Kurthen 2007)

Kurthen stresses several important ideas: he suggests that only through the embodied nature of the cognitive system internal states can acquire meaning (or significance); however, as he also points out, the "embodied action" approach alone does not yet solve the problems of the orthodoxy, because what is actually needed is an account of teleology. According to Kurthen, embodiment can only be a mediator, a "vehicle" of teleology. What needs to be considered is subsystems of the organism that support motivational and emotional states.

Under this conative view the functional subsystems of the organisms are to be rearranged. While most 'embodiment approaches' [...] stress the role of the sensorimotor system in embodied cognition, this system turns out to be of only secondary relevance from a teleological point of view. [...] Needs, desires and other conative states that fuel our actions are rooted in different parts of the organism: in the endocrine system, the autonomous nervous system and its target organs [...] as well as their regulatory centers in the brain stem (Kurthen 2007, 140)

The notion that cognition can only by understood by taking into account the organization and function of the body is also a key ingredient of the "sensorimotor contingency theory" (SCT) put forward by O'Regan and Noë (2001). According to SCT, the agent's sensorimotor contingencies, that is, the rules governing sensory changes produced by various motor actions, are constitutive for cognitive processes. "Seeing"—according to SCT—is not receiving an image on the retina, is not possessing a detailed internal "representation"; rather, seeing corresponds to knowing that one is currently engaged in a visual manipulation, in exploratory activity, mediated by knowledge of sensorimotor contingencies. The brain enables us to see, but the neural activity does not in itself constitute the seeing; rather, the brain supports vision by enabling exercise and mastery of sensorimotor contingencies. The SCT has interesting implications regarding the significance of internal states and neural activity patterns. I will return to this issue in the next section of this chapter. Another implication is that the concept of embodiment, as employed in the SCT and also in the other approaches I have mentioned, brings cognitive theory back to the personal level, i.e., a level where the acting system as a whole is described. Situatedness, then, also means bringing the cognitive system back into social context, an important perspective that can be unfolded in interesting ways following the pragmatic turn (cf. Mead 1934, 1938). For SCT, this would

TABLE 2
Key concepts of "pragmatic" cognitive science.

Primacy of action	Enactive view of cognition
Selection	Cognition as active, predictive process
Directives[a]	Implicit, partial, context-dependent encoding of contents
Self-Organization	Emphasis on intrinsic dynamics of cognitive systems
Decentralized cognition	Emergence in distributed architectures
Holism	Interaction (binding) of local processes/subsystems
Situatedness	Focus on embodiment and embeddedness into environment
Externalism	Cognitive system comprises both the agent and the ecological niche ("extended mind")

[a]The notion of a "directive" is introduced in Section 10.6 below and is meant to denote an anti-representationalist view of the significance of internal states of a cognitive system.

entail a generalization of the notion of "sensorimotor" contingencies to "action contingencies" and to "situations" as broader spatio-temporal contexts.

10.5   Action-Oriented View on Neural Processing

If we decide to go for a pragmatic turn in cognitive science, our view of the brain and its function are likely to change profoundly. The conceptual premises of the pragmatic stance can be mapped to the neuroscientific level of description and, thus, lead us to redefining at least some of the neurobiologist's explananda. What neuroscience, then, has to explain is not how brains act as world-mirroring devices, but how they can serve as "vehicles of world-making" that support, based on individual learning history, the construction of the experienced world and the guidance of action. The following premises might become part of a framework for "pragmatic neuroscience":

- The primary concern of the experimenter is not the relation of neural activity patterns to stimuli, but to the action at hand and the situation the subject under study is currently engaged in.
- The function of neural circuits has to be studied making reference to the view that cognition is a highly active, selective and constructive process.

- Sensory processing must be considered in a holistic perspective, as being subject to strong top-down influences that constantly create predictions about forthcoming sensory events and eventually reflect constraints from current action.
- The function of neurons and neural modules must not be considered in isolation, but with proper reference to contextual activity of other subsystems and the actions of the whole cognitive system.
- The investigation of the large-scale dynamics of the brain becomes increasingly important, since interactions within and across neural assemblies are constitutive of the operations of the cognitive system.
- Since the representational view is largely abandoned, a new view on the functional roles of neural states needs to be developed; rather than "encoding" information about pre-given objects or events in the world, neural states should be viewed as supporting the capacity of structuring situations that the agent is engaged in.

There is ample neurobiological evidence to suggest a fundamental role of action and of sensorimotor activity in perception and cognitive processing. In the following, I will briefly highlight some key findings that match the premises and predictions phrased above and, thus, seem to support a pragmatic stance for cognitive neuroscience.

Key evidence supporting the pragmatic view is provided by findings on the role of exploratory activity and sensorimotor interactions for neural development and plasticity. It has been known for a long time that developmental processes in the nervous system are activity-dependent. For instance, development of neural circuits in the visual system and acquisition of visuomotor skills critically depend on sensorimotor interactions and active exploration of the environment (cf. Held 1965, Majewska and Sur 2006). Even in the adult brain, there is considerable plasticity of cortical maps e.g., in the somatosensory and motor system that has been shown to depend on action context and, interestingly, also on attention (cf. Blake et al. 2002, Münte et al. 2002). Thus, for instance, after extensive practice with fingers 2, 3 and 4, monkeys acquire an increased number of tactile receptive fields on the respective fingertips; in the somatosensory cortex, the area receiving input from the trained fingers is enlarged (cf. Blake et al. 2002). Similar evidence is available for the human brain, e.g., in highly trained musicians who often show functional and structural changes in their sensorimotor system resulting from action-dependent plasticity (cf. Münte et al. 2002). One conclusion from these studies is that appropriate action, allowing exercise of relevant sensorimotor contingencies, is necessary throughout life to stabilize the functional architecture in the respective circuits.

Another important line of evidence concerns research on the function and neural mechanisms of "corollary discharge" or "reafference" signals, which are necessary for an organism to distinguish self-generated sensory changes from those not related to own action (cf. Desmurget and Grafton 2000). In technical contexts, the same principle is often referred to as a "forward model". Supporting the SCT, this research shows that predictions about the sensory outcome of movement are critical for the basic interpretation of sensory inputs. The importance of reafference has been shown in the context of eye movements and grasping or reaching movements. Interestingly, similar principles of predicting sensory inputs seem also to play a key role in more complex cognitive processes like language comprehension (cf. Pickering and Garrod 2006) or predictions about the actions of other subjects in social contexts (cf. Wilson and Knoblich 2005). A point of key interest is that in all these cases activity of motor planning regions seems involved in generating the prediction about sensory events, possibly by modulating neural signals in sensory regions (cf. Wilson and Knoblich 2005, Christensen et al. 2007). Malfunction of such modulatory signals and associated disturbance of forward models for predicting the consequences of own action have been implicated in the pathogenesis of psychiatric disorders such as schizophrenia (cf. Frith et al. 2000).

If guidance of action is a dominant function of the brain, one would predict that neuronal response profiles in sensory or association regions should strongly depend on action context. Indeed, there is clear evidence for such an action-relatedness. For instance, activation of visual neurons changes profoundly if unrestrained, self-induced eye movements are permitted, as compared to passive viewing of stimuli under controlled fixation (cf. Gallant et al. 1998). Furthermore, properties of parietal and premotor neurons strongly depend on action context (cf. Graziano and Gross 1998). In premotor cortex, the spatial profile of multimodal receptive fields depends on body and limb position (cf. Graziano et al. 1997). Tactile and visual receptive fields of premotor neurons are in dynamic register and seem "anchored" to body parts even if these are moving, suggesting that such polymodal neurons support predictions about expected changes in sensory input. Given the abundance of sensorimotor "gain" modulation of neural responses (cf. Salinas and Sejnowski 2001) and of dynamic sensorimotor interactions (cf. Engel et al. 2001), it seems likely that neural "representations" are always, to a considerable extent, action-related or action-modulated (cf. Clark 1997). In particular, it seems plausible to assume that neural assemblies (cf. Hebb 1949) supporting object-related knowledge are never purely sensory, but always correspond to large-scale multisensory and sensorimotor patterns with strong dependence on action context (cf. Johnson-Frey 2004).[10]

In the present context, another highly intriguing finding is that motor and premotor systems are also active during "virtual actions" (cf. Jeannerod 2001) like, for instance, "mental rotation" of objects (cf. Richter et al. 2000). Conversely, "virtual action" apparently can have a profound influence on experienced sensory structure. This is beautifully demonstrated by a study of Bisiach and Luzzatti (1978) in patients suffering from unilateral neglect due to damage in the right parietal cortex. The term "neglect" denotes a profound inability to access sensory information in peripersonal space contralateral to the lesion. Interestingly, in these patients neglect was also found under conditions of visual imagery: when asked to imagine known spatial settings, the patients could only report the right half of the respective scene; even more striking, when now the patient imagined turning by 180 degrees, she could suddenly access, in her imagination, the parts of the scene on the formerly neglected side. These observations on the relation between neglect and imagined action suggest a fundamental role of action planning centers in the modulation of complex cognitive processes.

Along the same lines, there is evidence for a role of premotor structures in directing attention and even in controlling the access of sensory signals to consciousness. Recent studies on neural mechanisms of attention clearly support a cognitive role of action-generating circuits (cf. Kastner and Ungerleider 2000). As part of what has been called a "premotor theory of attention" (Rizzolatti et al. 1987), it has long been suggested that the selection of sensory information should be modulated and focussed by constraints arising from current action planning and execution. In agreement with this prediction, several studies have shown that movement preparation can lead to attentional shifts and to changes in the acquisition of object-related information (cf. Craighero et al. 1999, Eimer and van Velzen 2006, Fagioli et al. 2007). Functional imaging studies in humans provide evidence that the modulatory bias imposed by attention may indeed arise from premotor regions (cf. Corbetta et al. 1998). In a recent study using an "attentional blink" paradigm, we have obtained evidence that a network of premotor, parietal and limbic regions modulates the dynamics of conscious visual processing (cf. Kranczioch et al. 2005). Moreover, in recent MEG

---

[10]It should be noted that the view expressed here differs substantially from the "theory of event coding" developed by Hommel et al. (2001). While this approach posits a fundamental unity of perception and action, the ideas it implies on "common coding" are restricted to high-level processing domains and are not applied to presumed "low-level" sensory and motor networks. I oppose the latter view.

experiments on visual attention we could show that premotor regions
like the frontal eye field are involved in top-down modulation of the
timing in sensory assemblies (cf. Siegel et al. 2008). Clearly, these findings support the premotor theory of attention.[11] Actually, these data
suggest that attention may be best understood as a bias in sensory
processing that arises from the informational needs imposed by current
or planned action.

10.6 Dismissing Representationalism

From the observations discussed above, one may conclude that the functional significance of neural states or activity patterns needs to be re-
defined, because a representational account eventually fails to provide
a satisfying view. As we have discussed above, neural patterns do not
carry "images" of the external world. What these patterns support are
not abstract structural descriptions of objects and scenes but, rather,
knowledge about sets of possible actions that produce viable segmen-
tations of the scene. Neural activity patterns, on this account, support
the organism's capacity of structuring situational contexts; they "prescribe" possible actions, rather than "describing" states of the outside
world. In fact, their functional role in the guidance of action is what
determines the "meaning" of internal states. Clark summarizes:

> [T]he brain should not be seen as primarily a locus of inner descriptions
> of external states of affairs; rather, it should be seen as a locus of
> inner structures that act as operators upon the world via their role in
> determining actions. (Clark 1997, 47)

The need to redefine the functional role of internal states has apparently been acknowledged by forerunners of the pragmatic turn who,
in different versions, made attempts to soften up the connotations of
the term "representation" by introducing additional qualifiers. To denote the action-relatedness of internal states and to emphasize that
objects and events of the current situation are specified with respect
to the cognitive agent, concepts like "deictic representation" (Chapman 1991), "indexical representation" (Agre 1997), "control-oriented
representation" (Clark 1995), "deictic codes" (Ballard et al. 1997) or

---

[11]The "premotor theory of attention" provides an example for the hypothesis
implied by the pragmatic, or enactive approach, that covert mental acts can possibly
be grounded in "simulated actions". In the premotor account, covert refocussing of
attention is understood as being closely related to overt orienting movement of eye,
head and body, and being a derivative of overt action. As demonstrated by the
studies cited in the main text, a lot is known about the brain structures involved
in attention, and the neural traces are essentially the same for overt and covert
attention.

"action-oriented representation" (Clark 1997) have been introduced. While all this is helpful, I think that these indecisive attempts to undermine the usage of the notion of "representation" can be recast in a slightly more radical way. It seems that the smarter move is to drop the term "representation" altogether and to replace it by an expression that does not carry about so much of the cognitivist burden.

I propose to use the notion of a *"directive"* rather than that of "representation" for characterizing the functioning of dynamic patterns of interactions in a cognitive system. Introducing this term as part of the pragmatic framework, it is important to stress that directives are not simply internal states of the brain. They are, of course, supported by neural activity patterns, but they correspond to states of the cognitive system in its entirety. Importantly, such action-oriented patterns will always include certain aspects of bodily dynamics, e.g., certain biophysical properties of the skeletomuscular system. Actually, they might best be described as *patterns of dynamic interactions extending through the entire cognitive system.* This is why "directive" is not just a different term for "action-oriented representation". The latter is "in the head", the former denotes the dynamics of the "extended mind" (cf. Clark 2008).

What, then, is the relation of directives to actions and objects on the one hand, and to neural states on the other? As proposed here, directives are immediately related to action selection. Activating directives directly controls the respective action. More generally, directives correspond to dispositions for meaningful actions; as such, they correspond to ways of "knowing-how" rather than "knowing-that".[12] Object concepts, then, correspond to sets of related directives; on this account, knowing what a glass or a tree is does not mean to possess internal descriptions of such objects, but to master sets of sensorimotor skills, paths of possible action that can be taken to explore or utilize the respective object. Objects are not "targeted by" directives but, rather, they are constituted by these because, in fact, an object is defined by the set of possible actions that can be performed on it. We do not first perceive a chair by setting up an abstract geometric description, and then compute its suitability for sitting; rather, perceiving a chair *is* to detect the opportunity of sitting. The concept of an object corresponds to "nothing but" the set of possible actions relating to this object; there is no context-neutral "description" above and beyond the direc-

---

[12]Indeed, an assumption implied in the pragmatic approach is that "knowing-how" is fundamental, and "knowing-that" a derived mode of knowledge; accordingly, "procedural" or "implicit" learning is basic, and other forms of learning are grounded in these.

tives.[13] The relation between directives and their neural underpinnings can be phrased as follows: Directives correspond to functional roles of neural states; conversely, neural activity patterns support and partially implement a directive's functional role. Thus, directives provide a network of functional roles, defined by current action, that are supported by dynamic patterns in neural activity. It is important to note that neural activity patterns are not directives themselves, but only their "traces" accessible to neurophysiological experimentation. The "neural vehicles" of directives, of course, can be assumed to be highly complex, very likely involving cell populations distributed across numerous regions of the brain.

10.7 Outlook

In this chapter I have—trying to build on recent developments in the field—introduced two concepts that might be useful in the discussion on how to create a *better* science of the mind. The first is the concept of a pragmatic turn, which denotes more of an agenda than a paradigm already in place. As should have become clear, the punch line is to eventually transform the whole theory of cognition into a theory of action. Notably, this is not a behaviorist move, since the dynamics of the cognitive system is at the very heart of the enterprise, and clear reference is made to "states in" the cognitive system. I have tried to show that an action-oriented framework is not only conceptually viable but, in fact, already supported by much experimental evidence. Numerous findings in neuroscience either overtly demonstrate the action-relatedness of cognitive processing, or can be re-interpreted more elegantly in this new framework. The second notion I have introduced is that of a "directive", which I nominate as a conceptual antagonist to the cognitivist notion of "representation". Future work will tell if my hypotheses on "directives" can be consolidated into a robust theory of the dynamics of cognitive systems.

In an earlier section of this chapter, I have been outlining how key assumptions may be changing in a "pragmatic neuroscience". As I mentioned, a key question is whether these conceptual shifts may eventually lead us to a different style of experimentation, to different settings and paradigms, to new laboratory habits. I think, they will and, actually, many harbingers have arrived and begin taking effect. More and more

---

[13]The view discussed here clearly bears some resemblance to the Gibsonian theory of affordances (cf. Gibson 1986). However, a critical difference is that Gibson sees affordances as observer-invariant features of objects. This does not hold for directives, which prescribe, or embody, patterns of actions in highly context-sensitive ways.

researchers in the field implicitly seem to set up their own prescriptions for a pragmatic cognitive science, starting to use natural stimuli, complex sensorimotor paradigms, massively parallel recording techniques and, most importantly, less restrained subjects. The fans of the pragmatic turn should be the first to realize that the return of the active cognizer to the lab is, above all, a matter of practice, rather than of theory.

Acknowledgements

This work has been supported by a grant from the Volkswagen Foundation (project "Representation").

References

Agre, P. 1997. *Computation and Human Experience*. Cambridge University Press.

Aloimonos, Y. and A. Rosenfeld. 1991. Computer vision. *Science* 253:1249–1254.

Ballard, D.H., M.M. Hayhoe, P.K. Pook, and R.P.N. Rao. 1997. Deictic codes for the embodiment of cognition. *Behavioral and Brain Sciences* 20:723–767.

Barlow, H.B. 1972. Single units and sensation: A neuron doctrine for perceptual psychology? *Perception* 1:371–394.

Bartels, A. and M. May. 2009. Functional role theories of representation and content explanation: with a case study from spatial cognition. *Cognitive Processing* 10:63–75.

Biederman, I. 1987. Recognition-by-components: a theory of human image understanding. *Psychological Review* 94:115–147.

Bisiach, E. and C. Luzzatti. 1978. Unilateral neglect of representational space. *Cortex* 14:129–133.

Blake, D.T., N.N. Byl, and M.M. Merzenich. 2002. Representation of the hand in the cerebral cortex. *Behavioural Brain Research* 135:179–184.

Brooks, R. 1991. Intelligence without representation. *Artificial Intelligence* 47:139–160.

Burge, T. 1979. Individualism and the mental. In P. French, T. Uehling, and H. Wettstein, eds., *Midwest Studies in Philosophy*, vol. IV, pages 73–121. University of Minnesota Press.

Chapman, D. 1991. *Vision, Instruction, and Action*. MIT Press.

Christensen, M.S., J. Lundbye-Jensen, S.S. Geertsen, T.H. Petersen, O.B. Paulson, and J.B. Nielsen. 2007. Premotor cortex modulates somatosensory cortex during voluntary movement without proprioceptive feedback. *Nature Neuroscience* 10:417–419.

Churchland, P.S., V.S. Ramachandran, and T.J. Sejnowski. 1994. A critique of pure vision. In C. Koch and J. Davis, eds., *Large-Scale Neuronal Theories of the Brain*, pages 23–60. MIT Press.

Churchland, P.S. and T.J. Sejnowksi. 1992. *The Computational Brain*. MIT Press.

Clancey, W.J. 1997. *Situated Cognition: On Human Knowledge and Computer Representations*. Cambridge University Press.

Clark, A. 1995. Moving minds: situating content in the service of real-time success. In J. Tomberlin, ed., *Philosophical Perspectives*, vol. 9 of *AI, Connectionism and Philosophical Psychology*, pages 89–104. Ridgeview.

Clark, A. 1997. *Being There. Putting Brain, Body, and World Together Again*. MIT Press.

Clark, A. 1999. An embodied cognitive science? *Trends in Cognitive Sciences* 3:345–351.

Clark, A. 2008. *Supersizing the Mind: Embodiment, Action and Cognitive Extension*. Oxford University Press.

Corbetta, M., E. Akbudak, T.E. Conturo, A.Z. Snyder, J.M. Ollinger, H.A. Drury, M.R. Linenweber, S.E. Petersen, M.E. Raichle, D.C. Van Essen, and G.L. Shulman. 1998. A common network of functional areas for attention and eye movements. *Neuron* 21:761–773.

Craighero, L., L. Fadiga, G. Rizzolatti, and C. Umilta. 1999. Action for perception: a motor-visual attentional effect. *Journal of Experimental Psychology: Human Perception and Performance* 25:1673–1692.

Cummins, R. 1996. *Representations, Targets, and Attitudes*. MIT Press.

Desmurget, M. and S. Grafton. 2000. Forward modelling allows feedback control for fast reaching movements. *Trends in Cognitive Sciences* 4:423–431.

Dewey, J. 1896. The reflex arc concept in psychology. *Psychological Review* 3:357–370.

Dewey, J. 1925. *Experience and Nature*. Open Court.

Dreyfus, H.L. 1992. *What Computers Still Can't Do*. MIT Press.

Eimer, M. and J. van Velzen. 2006. Covert manual response preparation triggers attentional modulations of visual but not auditory processing. *Clinical Neurophysiology* 117:1063–1074.

Engel, A.K., P. Fries, and W. Singer. 2001. Dynamic predictions: oscillations and synchrony in top-down processing. *Nature Reviews Neuroscience* 2:704–716.

Engel, A.K. and P. König. 1998. Paradigm shifts in the neurobiology of perception. In U. Ratsch, M. Richter, and I.-O. Stamatescu, eds., *Intelligence and Artificial Intelligence. An Interdisciplinary Debate*, pages 178–192. Springer.

Fagioli, S., B. Hommel, and R.I. Schubotz. 2007. Intentional control of attention: action planning primes action-related stimulus dimensions. *Psychological Research* 71:22–29.

Findlay, J.M. and I.D. Gilchrist. 2003. *Active Vision. The Psychology of Looking and Seeing*. Oxford University Press.

Fodor, J.A. 1987. *Psychosemantics: The Problem of Meaning in the Philosophy of Mind*. MIT Press.

Fodor, J.A. 1990. *A Theory of Content and Other Essays*. MIT Press.

Fodor, J.A. and Z.W. Pylyshyn. 1988. Connectionism and cognitive architecture: a critical analysis. *Cognition* 28:3–71.

Frith, C.D., S.-J. Blakemore, and D.M. Wolpert. 2000. Explaining the symptoms of schizophrenia: abnormalities in the awareness of action. *Brain Research Reviews* 31:357–363.

Gallant, J.L., C.E. Connor, and D.C. Van Essen. 1998. Neural activity in areas V1, V2 and V4 during free viewing of natural scenes compared to controlled viewing. *Neuroreport* 9:85–89.

Gibson, J.J. 1986. *The Ecological Approach to Visual Perception*. Lawrence Erlbaum.

Graziano, M.S.A. and C.G. Gross. 1998. Spatial maps for the control of movement. *Current Opinion in Neurobiology* 8:195–201.

Graziano, M.S.A., X.T. Hu, and C.G. Gross. 1997. Visuospatial properties of ventral premotor cortex. *Journal of Neurophysiology* 77:2268–2292.

Hebb, D.O. 1949. *The Organization of Behavior*. Wiley.

Heidegger, M. 1986. *Sein und Zeit*. Niemeyer.

Heidegger, M. 1989. *Die Grundprobleme der Phänomenologie*. Klostermann.

Held, R. 1965. Plasticity in sensory-motor systems. *Scientific American* 11(65):84–94.

Hommel, B., J. Müsseler, G. Aschersleben, and W. Prinz. 2001. The theory of event coding (TEC): a framework for perception and action planning. *Behavioral and Brain Sciences* 24:849–937.

Hubel, D.H. 1988. *Eye, Brain, and Vision*. Freeman.

Jeannerod, M. 2001. Neural simulation of action: a unifying mechanism for motor cognition. *Neuroimage* 14:S103–S109.

Johnson-Frey, S.H. 2004. The neural basis of complex tool use in humans. *Trends in Cognitive Sciences* 8:71–78.

Kastner, S. and L.G. Ungerleider. 2000. Mechanisms of visual attention in the human cortex. *Annual Review of Neuroscience* 23:315–341.

Kranczioch, C., S. Debener, J. Schwarzbach, R. Goebel, and A.K. Engel. 2005. Neural correlates of conscious perception in the attentional blink. *NeuroImage* 24:704–714.

Kurthen, M. 1992. *Neurosemantik. Grundlagen einer praxiologischen kognitiven Neurowissenschaft*. Enke.

Kurthen, M. 1994. *Hermeneutische Kognitionswissenschaft*. Djre Verlag.

Kurthen, M. 2007. From mind to action: the return of the body in cognitive science. In S. Sielke and E. Schäfer-Wünsche, eds., *The Body as Interface: Dialogues Between the Disciplines*, pages 129–143. Winter Verlag.

Majewska, A.K. and M. Sur. 2006. Plasticity and specificity of cortical processing networks. *Trends in Neurosciences* 29:323–329.

Marr, D. 1982. *Vision*. Freeman.

Mead, G.H. 1934. *Mind, Self and Society*. University of Chicago Press.

Mead, G.H. 1938. *The Philosophy of the Act*. University of Chicago Press.

Merleau-Ponty, M. 1962. *Structure of Behaviour*. Beacon Press.

Merleau-Ponty, M. 1963. *Phenomenology of Perception*. Humanities Press.

Münte, T.F., E. Altenmüller, and L. Jäncke. 2002. The musician's brain as a model of neuroplasticity. *Nature Reviews Neuroscience* 3:473–478.

Newell, A. and H.A. Simon. 1976. Computer science as empirical enquiry: Symbols and search. *Communications of the Association for Computing Machinery* 19:113–126.

Noë, A. 2004. *Action in Perception*. MIT Press.

Noë, A. 2009. *Out of Our Heads*. Hill and Wang.

O'Regan, J.K. and A. Noë. 2001. The sensorimotor account of vision and visual consciousness. *Behavioural and Brain Sciences* 24:939–1031.

Palmer, S.E. 1999. *Vision Science*. MIT Press.

Pickering, M.J. and S. Garrod. 2006. Do people use language production to make predictions during comprehension? *Trends in Cognitive Sciences* 11:105–110.

Rey, G. 1997. *Contemporary Philosophy of Mind: A Contentiously Classical Approach*. Blackwell.

Richter, W., R. Somorjai, R. Summers, M. Jarmasz, R.S. Menon, J.S. Gati, A.P. Georgopoulos, C. Tegeler, K. Ugurbil, and S.G. Kim. 2000. Motor area activity during mental rotation studied by time-resolved single-trial fMRI. *Journal of Cognitive Neuroscience* 12:310–320.

Rizzolatti, G., L. Riggio, I. Dascola, and C. Umiltá. 1987. Reorienting attention across the horizontal and vertical meridians: evidence in favor of a premotor theory of attention. *Neuropsychologia* 25:31–40.

Salinas, E. and T.J. Sejnowski. 2001. Gain modulation in the central nervous system: where behaviour, neurophysiology, and computation meet. *Neuroscientist* 7:430–440.

Siegel, M., T.H. Donner, R. Oostenveld, P. Fries, and A.K. Engel. 2008. Neuronal synchronization along the dorsal visual pathway reflects the focus of spatial attention. *Neuron* 60:709–719.

Ullman, S. 1991. Tacit assumptions in the computational study of vision. In A. Gorea, ed., *Representations of Vision*, pages 305–317. Cambridge University Press.

Varela, F.J., E. Thompson, and E. Rosch. 1991. *The Embodied Mind. Cognitive Science and Human Experience*. MIT Press.

Wilson, M. and G. Knoblich. 2005. The case for motor involvement in perceiving conspecifics. *Psychological Bulletin* 131:460–473.

Winograd, T. and F. Flores. 1986. *Understanding Computers and Cognition*. Ablex Publishing.

Index

general purpose, 213
-how, *see* knowing-how
implicit, 90, 92–94
non-propositional, *see*
    knowing-how
perceptual, 93
practical, 79, 84, 94–96, 101,
    103
procedural, 90
propositional, *see* knowing-that
tacit, 31, 36, 91–92
-that, *see* knowing-that
theoretical, 79, 80, 82, 94–96,
    103
visual, 97
visually guided, 93
knowledge format, 79, 96–101,
    103
image-like, 79, 96–103
propositional, 79, 96–103
sensorimotor, 79, 96–103
knowledge problem, 124, 125
"knowledge representation"
    project, 85, 86, 90–94, 96, 103

Language of Thought, *see* LOT
LOT, 26, 31–34, 36, 37, 41, 42,
    45–49, 94, 96

M-intention, 102
malfunction, 173, 181, *see also*
    representation,
    misrepresentation; content,
    normal conditions
map
    cortical, 223
Marr, David, 180, 213
Mead, George H., 217
mechanism, *see also* explanation,
    mechanistic
activity, 165–168
basic, 131, 143*fn*
causal, 180*fn*
complex, 91, 145

component, 137, 139–141,
    141*fn*, 143–145, 150, 165,
    166, 168, 182
composition, 164, 165
feed-back, 115, 118, 122, 136,
    144, 145, 145*fig*, 146, 154,
    155, 174
functional decomposition, 145,
    165, *see also* analysis,
    functional
information processing, 129,
    164, 182
intercellular, 146
intracellular, 146
linkage, 135, 137, 138
neural, 224
operation, 136–140, 140*fn*, 141,
    143–146, 150, 165, 166
organization, 137, 146, 164, 165
recomposition, 145
regulation of, 140–142
simple, 203
simple localization, 143, 143*fn*,
    144, 145
structural decomposition, 144,
    145, 165
Merleau-Ponty, Maurice, 215,
    217–219
Millikan, Ruth G., 121*fn*, 130,
    131*fn*, 138*fn*, 169, 187, 188*fn*,
    189, 190, 192, 194
misrepresentation, *see*
    representation,
    misrepresentation
model, 114, 119, 145*fn*, 193,
    195–197, 197*fn*, 198, **198**,
    200, *see also* representation,
    isomorphism;
    –homomorphism
forward, 224
mechanical, 119
mental, 197*fn*, 200
neurophysiological, 214*tab*
world-model, 211, 213, 214, 219
motor cortex, 33